AF539742

Clinical Psychology

New Trends and Innovations

Clinical Psychology

New Trends and Innovations

RAJPAL KAUR

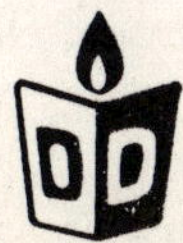

DEEP & DEEP PUBLICATIONS PVT. LTD.
F-159, Rajouri Garden, New Delhi - 110 027

CLINICAL PSYCHOLOGY

ISBN 81-7629-801-8

Printed in India at NEW ELEGANT PRINTERS,
A-49/1, Mayapuri, Phase-I, New Delhi - 110 064.

Published by DEEP & DEEP PUBLICATIONS PVT. LTD.,
F-159, Rajouri Garden, New Delhi - 110 027 • Phone : 25435369, 25440916
E-mail : deep98@del3.vsnl.net.in • ddpbooks@yahoo.co.in
Showroom :
2/13, Ansari Road, Daryaganj, New Delhi - 110 002 • Telefax : 23245122

Contents

Preface

Clinical psychology is the application of psychology within a clinical (health) setting. However, it is often taken to refer primarily to the easing of psychological distress, mental illness or mental health problems. The term was introduced in a 1907 paper by the American psychologist Lightner Witmer (1867-1956).

Clinical psychologists are involved in the diagnosis, assessment, and treatment of patients with psychiatric disorders, as well as research about all of these areas of clinical practice. Their clinical work may include the use of 'talk therapies' (i.e., psychotherapy such as cognitive therapy and psychoanalysis), or the use of psychological tests to assess certain aspects of psychological functioning.

Some clinical psychologists may specialize in understanding, assessing, and treating brain injury and neurocognitive deficits to become clinical neuropsychologists.

Prior to the 20th century, there was little, if any, clinical help available for sufferers of mental health problems. In the early 20th century, Sigmund Freud developed a therapy known as psychoanalysis. The practice of psychoanalysis was initially restricted to psychiatrists (medical doctors who specialise in treating mental illness) but is currently practiced by psychologists and other mental health practitioners. Psychoanalytic training is a lengthy endeavour, often taking the analytic candidate, who is already a psychologist or psychiatrist, an additional five to ten years to complete.

Clinical psychology developed partly as a result of a need for additional clinicians to treat mental health problems, and partly as psychological science advanced to the stage where the fruits of psychological research could be successfully applied in clinical settings.

The field of clinical psychology is an extremely complex one, and moving about in it with ease and assurance requires a breadth of understanding that is not easily attained. It is therefore not surprising to find that a clear pathway of progressive study has not been provided for the student of clinical psychology. In some instances the student begins a formal course in the clinical field with no more background than that provided by a single course in general psychology, while in other instances no formal course is provided until the student is well along in a graduate program.

The books available to the student are either specialized manuals for the clinician or books devoted to measurement or evaluation. The present book, recognizing these facts, represents an effort to present a systematic and integrated group of topics that are fundamental to satisfactory movement in the clinical field. The emphasis of the book is placed on theory and methodology and is therefore directed both to the beginning student in clinical psychology and to the person who has developed some competence with clinical techniques. For the beginning student the book should serve as an introduction to later training and practice. We have assumed that such a student will have some knowledge of general and abnormal psychology. In an ideal situation, of course, he would have broad basic preparation. For the advanced student the book will tie together the personality and clinical field in such a way as to give his procedures more meaning.

This text is not designed to serve as a clinical manual. Competence in clinical practice demands much more than a book. It depends upon direct experience, broad reading, a deep understanding of human nature, constant attention to the latest research. Nor is the book set up for a full description of the special procedures and techniques. These have been provided in many other sources, a bibliography of which has been included.

The emphasis has, instead, been placed on basic principles, methodology, and general techniques. This emphasis should provide the foundation necessary for growth in proficiency and for more complete understanding of the administration and interpretation of the technical instruments of diagnosis and the methods of conducting a therapeutic interview. The book encourages the student to become something more than a technician who administers and interprets tests and helps him to develop a greater responsibility for making progress in the development of knowledge and procedures. The reader is urged persistently to develop the critical faculty which is so badly needed in the clinical field because of the tentative and often confused nature of so many of its concepts. We have tried to write a critical and hard-headed account of the clinical area, and at the same time put across an appreciation for the sounder principles and for the methodological problems we face as clinical psychologists.

I am grateful to all who have cooperated in finalising this book. I acknowledge with thanks the help of various librarians and authors of various books which have been referred to in this book. I would also like to thank the publishers for bringing this book out in time.

RAJPAL KAUR

1

Clinical Psychology: Definition and Meaning

Introduction

A psychologist reading contemporary journal literature is being influenced unknowingly by an editorial decision that took place not too many years ago. The sheer productivity of the increased number of psychologists forced editors to eliminate or drastically curtail what at one time was an essential part of the research report-the historical introduction. Today, the first rule of article writing is to come immediately to the point. The setting for this point is often limited to no more than, "Since Brown has found that then, or the immortal phrase, "In a previous communication. It is not surprising then that readers, especially among younger psychologists, may slip into thinking that this work began with "Brown" or with the "previous communication," since this is the only work cited. Thus a valuable source of historical perspective has been lost, with no foreseeable chance that the custom will change. In the master's essay and the doctoral dissertation some attempt is still made to place a research problem in its historical context, but the value of these attempts is blunted by the sponsors' injunction to students; "When you prepare for publication, the first thing to eliminate is the historical introduction."

The change of policy about historical introductions may be both an effect of an a historical, or even anti-historical, attitude on the part of psychologists and one of the causes of the continued neglect of history.

This foreshortening of historical vision is perhaps one of the reasons that clinical psychologists are, to a considerable, degree, blithely oblivious to much of the content of experimental psychology on which their clinical efforts are based. The breach between "experimental" and "clinical" psychologists is obviously widened if no attempt is made to show that they are related. One of the sources of furthering rapprochement between these factions is attention to the historical antecedents of clinical work to be found in non clinical settings.

Looking at historically rooted experimental antecedents of clinical psychology is a process similar to the clinical investigation of the investigation of the individual. A psychological problem viewed both in present context, as it is in the chapters to follow, and in historical perspective, as it is in this chapter, is like viewing the patient as reflecting both contemporary forces and past experiences. Most clinical psychologists, in attempting to understand a patient's current problem, feel that they need to know the individual's past history; so too should we be sensitive to the need for understanding current research in the light of its historical antecedents.

Traditions of Clinical Psychology

The history of psychology shows a cumulative advance by the building up of a body of research findings, theories, procedures, and techniques which are passed on from one generation of psychologists to the next. Because of this passage between generations it is proper to speak of a tradition of psychology. Within this general tradition, it is possible to discern several more specific traditions, each not completely separable and tending to blend one with another, but sufficiently distinguishable so that they have come to receive meaningful identifying labels.

As a field, clinical psychology originated in a matrix of older, already existing traditions within psychology. Indeed no tradition of psychology is so remote from clinical endeavor as to be ruled out completely as one of the foundations of clinical psychology. Discernible among these as particularly relevant to clinical psychology are the psychometric, the dynamic, the social, the biological-medical, and the experimental traditions.

The intent of this book requires that the experimental tradition be made central. Some of the other traditions are peripheral to this emphasis. What is meant by these traditions is already familiar. In a Presidential Address to the American Psychological Association, Cronbach focused on the contrast between experimental psychology and what he called correlation psychology. He was in fact contrasting the experimental and psychometric traditions. Bindra and Scheier , who wrote on the relation between what they called psychometric and experimental research, were also considering these two traditions. Omitted from this chapter is the psychiatric tradition as it is reflected, in the immediate past, in the field of the study of individual differences, stemming from Galton and Cattell, and the effect of this study upon psychology in general and upon clinical psychology in particular. This omission is justified, not because the study of individual differences is unimportant, but because it is sufficiently separable from the experimental tradition in the direction of the psychometric tradition to justify omission. The absence of much material on the human child illustrates this point, since so much research using children is dependent upon the use of already established differences. Some aspects of the psychometric tradition are discussed in the chapter by Berg on measurement and evaluation.

Clinical psychology also draws upon the dynamic tradition, epitomized in the work of Freud, James, Hall and Janet. In a previous publication the writer explored historically the psychometric and dynamic tradition of clinical psychology. It is convenient to refer to the biological-medical tradition in psychology as a more or less coherent, interrelated whole. Not only does this draw attention to the fact that medical research is rooted in biology, making them for present purposes essentially one, but it also serves to distinguish it from medicine's contributions to the dynamic tradition.

The social tradition, drawing unto itself social philosophy, sociology, and social psychology (as well as experimental and clinical psychology), is, in itself, a hybrid similar in this respect to clinical psychology. Insofar as these traditions draw upon experiment they are relevant to that which follows. Their rich contextual and theoretical heritage as well as their use of other methodologies must be neglected.

Each of these other traditions has a symbiotic relation with clinical psychology. Each tradition supplies content and approaches to the clinical field and receives in return content and procedures, but here attention is centered on the contribution from the experimental field. The reverse relation is another story.

Implicit in the title of this book is the contention that clinical psychological research has as one of its bases the contributions of experimental behavioral study. In this sense the entire history of experimental psychology bears relation to clinical psychology. No attempt has been made in this volume to limit the experimental tradition to a narrow definition. Rather, experimental psychology was interpreted as behavioral study oriented to and derived from the laboratory but not confined to it, providing that the concern in non laboratory settings attempted to preserve, insofar as the problem and setting permitted, the controls of the laboratory. Despite the broad context of the entire book, however, it would be absurd to try in the space of a few pages to sketch the history of experimental psychology.

This chapter instead presents selected historical material in settings that will bring out their contemporary significance. The illustrations used are drawn from the experimental tradition particularly relevant to some of the major problems discussed in later chapters. Selection of each topic was guided by its usefulness not only as an illustration of historical relationships as such but also by its capacity to deepen the value of knowledge of the history of psychology. Knowledge, for example, that contemporary investigation of clinical judgment is rooted in the very oldest of problems in the experimental tradition, that of psychophysics, helps us to understand the significance of the research and to gain some understanding of the direction it has taken. Moreover the possibility of showing that psychophysics which occupies one of the highest floors in the Ivory Tower is relevant to clinical psychology is a temptation that could not be resisted.

Clinical Psychology and The Experimental Tradition in The Past

Clinical psychology, as a separate discipline, arose some time after the turn of the century. This approximate date is used to differentiate its past from its historical period.

This past stretched back in time to the earliest known experimentally controlled research study of the Ancient World. In fact, the earliest psychological experiment known to the writer is relevant to the topic of this Chapter, which is concerned with the effects of early experience on later behavior. As told by Herodotus, one Psammetichus, ruler of Egypt in the seventh century before Christ, wanted to enhance Egyptian national pride by proving that Egyptian was the oldest of languages. Accordingly, he ordered his herdsman to take two children "of the common sort" and to isolate them from birth onward in a hut, accompanied only by goats from which to draw nourishment; further, he gave strict instructions that no human beings be allowed to approach them. Two years later, when the hut was opened, the children rushed out crying, "becos." To the Pharaoh's chagrin, "becos" proved to be the Phrygian word for bread, forcing him to acknowledge that this, not Egyptian, was the oldest of languages.

To return to the period more than 2500 years later than Psammetichus-a considerable number of psychologists and other research workers can be considered possible early representatives of the experimental tradition in psychology. Some contributed so much to the intellectual climate of their times and influenced our own so forcefully that attention is forced upon them, despite the fact that they did their work before there was a clinical psychology. Representative of these are Darwin and Pavlov, towering above the others, who did not work with clinical problems and were, in fact, not even psychologists. But their contributions were so far reaching that they must be considered. Others, not so important, did experimental work which had direct relation with clinical problems, both in the past before clinical psychology emerged as a discipline and after the turn of the century when clinical psychology was beginning to emerge. By definition they were not clinical psychologists. Rather, they were individuals who contributed materially to experimental psychology but did so using clinical problems. Emil Kraepelin is representative of the past; Shepard Ivory Franz is representative of the period of emergence of clinical psychology.

Charles Darwin

Darwin was not the first biologist to concern himself with evolution. During the first half of the nineteenth century and even before, evolutionary theory excited considerable interest and furious discussion. Darwin's genius rested not upon proposing the problem, but upon his long and painstaking collection of the relevant evidence. The period of preparation began in 1831 with the voyage of H.M.S. "Beagle" to the South Seas, lasted through the years of travel, and culminated with his reading of Malthus's Essay on Population in 1838. Thereafter he had a biological premise to work with and his own theory of evolution began to take shape in the doctrine of the transmutation of the species. Over the next twenty years he collected the necessary mass of relevant data. Only in 1859 did On the Origin of Species appear. What happened thereafter, we can assume, is generally familiar. We need be concerned only with Darwin's effect on psychology; there, his The Expression of the Emotions in Man and Animals was important.

For the remainder of the century, psychology clearly evidenced the influence of Darwin. His work shaped psychology in the direction of biology and function and away from the model of physics and chemistry and structure of the German psychologists. One facet of the biological orientation, as a matter of fact, was the line of development, from Galton through Baldwin and Hall, in the study of individual differences. Evidences of this biological orientation were manifested in other ways as well. A sign of Darwin's influence was found in the increasing tendency to interpret mental processes in terms of the functions they served. Moreover, the comparative viewpoint of a continuity of mental development became prominent because of his work. It has even been suggested by Beck and Molish that to Darwin we owe the beginning of "scientific clinical psychology." They reach this conclusion because of his recognition of the importance of the dynamics of behavior. These trends in the work of those influenced by Darwin will be apparent in later discussion.

It was Darwin's work that stimulated the study of comparative psychology immediately prior to the modern era. For some years after Darwin the anecdotal method, dependent upon casual observation of "clever" and unusual animals, was the dominating technique for collecting data. This inadequate method was accompanied by a tendency to anthropomorphize the lower animals. About 1890 the work of Jacques Loeb and C. Lloyd Morgan introduced the modern era in animal psychology. Loeb's work on tropisms helped to demolish the trend toward anthropomorphism. So too did Morgan's canon, which might be stated briefly as advancing the rule that no action should be interpreted as being due to a higher behavioral function if it is capable of being interpreted as the outcome of a behavioral function lower in the scale. This adaptation of the law of parsimony served to discourage extravagant interpretation of animal behavior.

Ivan P. Pavlov

In his autobiography, Pavlov acknowledged that he was enormously influenced by Darwin, first through the intermediary of Pisarev's expositions of Darwin and the theory of evolution (Pisarev was a Russian writer of the sixties and seventies) and later directly by Darwin's works. The second major influence he acknowledged was the writings of Sechenov, whom he called the "father" of Russian physiology.

Through his researches Sechenov had become convinced that spinal reflexes are capable of inhibition by the cerebral cortex. He further argued that thinking and intelligence were dependent upon exercise for their stimulation and that all psychological acts are reflexes. As Pavlov indicated, Sechenov's view was based on conjecture. Pavlov proceeded to carry out his well-known research studies to demonstrate the validity of this hypothesis.

Pavlov acknowledged that Thorndike's researches of 1898 were the first experiments in this general area, but he further indicated that at the time he began investigation he was not familiar with this work.

Before embarking on the study of conditioning, a detailed study of the digestive glands had occupied a considerable amount of his research time. While working on these glands, Pavlov noticed that gastric juice was secreted by his experimental dogs not only when food was taken in the mouth but also when they saw it at a distance. Later on he found the same phenomena with the secretion of saliva. This "mouth watering" he first termed "psychical secretions," to distinguish this action-at-a-distance from direct stimulation of the nerve endings in the mouth. Heretofore, and indeed in his own early work, this and similar phenomena were considered in the then-current setting of introspective interpretation. The animal "judged" that it was food, that it "smelled good," and that he "desired" it. Pavlov's great contribution was to forego this introspective approach and treat the phenomena objectively. In other words, external stimulation and underlying nervous processes were studied experimentally by objective means. Pavlov followed this course by working on conditioned reflexes for his remaining thirty-five years.

His method, it should be noted, is extraordinarily flexible and has had far-reaching consequences. The conditioning referred to in later chapters, although perhaps initiated by problems quite alien to his range of interests, nevertheless all owe a debt to this physiologist. Vladimir Bechterev, too, beginning about 1907, studied the conditioning of motor responses. Bechterev 's work stimulated John B. Watson's enthusiastic presidential address in 1915, which was devoted to the topic of conditioning. However, as Hilgard and Marquis indicate, it was Pavlov's detailed approach to conditioning, not Bechterev's, which was accepted in the United States.

Emil Kraepelin

Born in 1856, Emil Kraepelin took a medical degree and subsequently was Professor of Psychiatry, first at Heidelberg and then at Munich. He is quite properly judged one of the founders of modern psychiatry-and sometimes described as the "father of descriptive psychiatry." This, in some circles, is dangerously close to epithet. What such critics forget is that his work on the classification and description of mental disorders made it possible for his successors to go further. Kraepelin himself seems to have been aware that it was too early to attempt more than description, for one of his papers ends expressly on the note that, once we have more knowledge, one can proceed to the main task-understanding the disorder.

He opened the first issue of his journal, Psychologische Arbeiten with an account of his own previous researches. He then proceeded to write eloquently that the psychological experiment is not merely useful but indispensable. He indicated that every psychiatrist seemed to judge it his right, or, perhaps even his obligation, to construct his own psychological system and went on to ask what internist would dare to proclaim a new system of physiology without basing it on a laboriously acquired laboratory fact? All of this has a modern ring; it was written more than sixty-five years ago but might still be pertinent today as comment and question.

Nevertheless, because his contributions to descriptive psychiatry were so immense, other facets of his work, of more direct concern to psychiatry, are often neglected, and it is seldom pointed out that experimental laboratory research was a major interest to Kraepelin.

Wundt had taken over the word association technique from Galton, and several of his students, including Kraepelin, worked in this area. On the heels of Cattell's first work on reaction time, Kraepelin showed that characteristic alterations in association occurred when experimentally induced abnormal conditions, such as fatigue, hunger, and alcoholic intoxication, were introduced. Another area in which Kraepelin was a pioneer was the study of continuous work, such as adding. He was able to show the classic phenomena-the shape of the curve, the mutually opposing influence of fatigue and learning, warming-up, spurts, and so on-which were nearly always found in subsequent investigations.

Shepard Ivory Franz

A physician, Edward Cowles, founded at McLean Hospital the first psychological laboratory for the investigation of psychotic patients. A charter member of the American Psychological Association in 1892, Cowles became director of the McLean Hospital some years before the turn of the century.

In 1903 Cowles invited psychologist Shepard Ivory Franz to come to the hospital laboratory to carry out some research that earlier he had asked Franz to outline. This work had to do with relating the nerve physiology that Sherrington was then developing to problems of excitement and depression as formulated by Kraepelin. In 1907 after carrying out this research, Franz went to what is now St.

Elizabeths Hospital in Washington, D.C., the federal mental hospital. He also had an appointment at George Washington University. His first task was to prepare a standard clinical psychological examination, adopted for use in the hospital in 1907 and expanded into a book, first published in 1912. This was almost certainly the first routine psychological examination program in the world. However, his work in the experimental tradition is more relevant to the present interest.

Before going to McLean Hospital, Franz, a Cattell Ph.D. from Columbia, had published his first paper in the field with which he was to become identified. This was the study entitled, "On the function of the cerebrum: the frontal lobes in relation to the production and retention of simple sensory-motor habits". His years at St. Elizabeths were productive in various fields. He studied, for example, the knee jerk in paretics. However, probably his most important work continued to have to do with cerebral function, especially in subjects in which brain areas were destroyed, and he published a considerable number of studies. Associated with him was Karl S. Lashley, and in 1917 they published together on the effects of cerebral destruction on habit formation in the white rat. From this point on the distinguished research work of Lashley continued along the lines thus laid down. Among his other younger associates was E. G. Boring, who spent the summer of 1913 with him, working in learning (and introspection) in dementia praecox.

Franz was by no means the only psychologist concerned with the abnormal person during these years. In a review of the experimental literature on psychotics through 1934 J. McV. Hunt reported on a considerable number of studies. After eliminating those irrelevant to present interests, such as psychometric and statistical studies, there were still about fifty experimental studies published before 1920. Among the other workers cited who used experimental methods with the psychotics before 1920 were J. W. Baird, A. Hoch, Grace H. Kent, T. V. Moore, E. W. Scripture, E. K. Strong, D. Wechsler, and F. L. Wells. Even this brief summary disproves the notion sometimes expressed that experimental study of the abnormal person was not taken seriously until more recent years.

Clinical Problems and The Experimental Tradition

At this point, the approach of this chapter shifts to consider historically some of the major themes of the topics to follow. It is manifestly impossible in short compass to trace, one by one, the historical backgrounds for the topics of the chapters that follow. Instead, the general headings of the sections, each including several chapters, supply the remaining topics; the first of these is divided into two parts. The topic of psychophysiology is not discussed specifically since in considerable measure it draws upon the biological-medical tradition. Insofar as psychophysiology draws upon learning, that section is relevant. The topics, then, are learning, communication, and behavior modification.

Learning

In the nineteenth century some of the previously mentioned animal research of Morgan and Loeb, as well as that of Faber, Lubbock, and Verworn, was experimental in intent, but it was Edward L. Thorndike who introduced the modern laboratory type of experiment into animal psychology. Beginning in 1898, his pioneer studies of learning and imitation in chicks, dogs, cats, and monkeys began to appear. Work similar in spirit immediately became popular among psychologists. The animal work of Yerkes, Carr, and Hunter during the first twenty-five years of this century is illustrative. However, it was John B. Watson who made the most far-reaching innovations in his popularization of behaviorism.

Before dealing with his work, it is necessary to say something about functional psychology, which was a characteristic expression of psychology in the United States during the early years of the century. Many factors were at work in its development. There was, for example, the influence of James from the United States and Hoffding and Kulpe from Europe. Another important factor was certainly the Darwinian influence. At the risk of some oversimplification, it will be this influence that will be sketched.

It was through functional psychology that the Darwinian view extended beyond animal psychology to psychology in general. The philosopher of social change, John Dewey, was influential in developing the functional point of view. As Boring demonstrates, he had been influenced by Darwinian thinking. The paper by Dewey published in 1896 with the self-explanatory title, "The reflex arc concept in psychology," had considerable influence. After Dewey's simultaneous departure from the University of Chicago (for Columbia University) and from psychology (for philosophy), his work was carried on by Angell. Angell, too, acknowledged a direct debt to Darwin, arguing that functional psychology was not new but had its modem impetus from the views of Darwin and Spencer (who also wrote in an evolutionary vein). As a "school," functionalism was relatively short-lived, and need not concern us further.

To return to Watson, who was trained at Chicago: much of the emphasis of functionalism lived on in behaviorism and in the neo behavioristic tendency, so prevalent today, to stress activity as contrasted with conscious states. Nevertheless, in one way functionalism strengthened Watson's rebellion-in this respect he was reacting as much against functionalism as against structuralism-in that functionalism, too, made no "clean break" with consciousness, and it was this break for which Watson argued. Watson himself stated that his debt was to C. Lloyd Morgan and Thorndike. The influence of Bechterev and Pavlov on Watson has already been mentioned. Watson began to formulate his views conversationally in 1903, gave them first public expression in 1905 to 1912, and first published them in 1913. Human behavior, learned and unlearned, with vigorous exclusion of introspective material, became a dominating force in American psychology under the enthusiastic sponsorship of Watson from about 1913 onward.

As behaviorism broadened, in the 1930's, from a school to a point of view without a school's in group manifestations, the next important figure to appear on the psychological scene was Clark L. Hull. In his autobiography Hull indicates how he came to his study of the quantitative laws of human behavior. He attributed his interest to his early training in the physical sciences; to being influenced favorably by Watson, although repelled by his dogmatism; and to reading Pavlov's Conditioned Reflexes, which had been translated in the late twenties. He goes on to indicate that about 1930 (after a considerable number of years of research endeavor on other problems) he came to the conclusion that the task of psychology as a natural science was the development of a "moderate" number of primary laws expressible quantitatively by means of ordinary equations, with the complex behavior of individuals to be derivable as secondary laws. His seminar became popular at the Institute of Human Relations at Yale University. Students, notably Kenneth W. Spence and Neal E. Miller, discussed this point of view with him, shared the general view, and conducted research along the lines laid down by Hull.

Of Hull's students Spence continued his work most directly; in a recent series of books surveying the present situation in psychology as a science a chapter is entitled, "The Hull-Spence Approach". The work of Spence is highly systematic and detailed. He insists, more than did Hull, upon holding his theorizing more closely to the research data, extending his views only as new data become available. His general attitude, his techniques, and his methods are summarized in an article which shows by its title, his allegiance to a modified behaviorism.

Spence's collaborative studies with Janet A. Taylor serve to illustrate another historical point: sometimes the experimental foundations of clinical psychology are to be found in contemporary research which precedes the clinically significant research by only a few years. For example, Taylor and Spence, initiating their studies on the relation of manifest anxiety and learning, first reported on them in 1952 and 1953. Taylor estimated that papers using the Manifest Anxiety Scale, published from 1952 through 1960, numbered about 300. Of these, 90 to 100 are quite directly concerned with the drive theory as proposed by Taylor and Spence. Their interest is and has been primarily in the role of drive in certain learning situations. Nevertheless, the extension of their work to the study of the phenomena of anxiety has also stimulated clinically oriented research-for example, that on the relationship of anxiety to stress.

Neal E. Miller, too, played an extensive role in the S-R reinforcement interpretation of learning. He has taken leadership in extending Hull's general point of view to approach-avoidance conflict behavior to psychotherapy and to social behavior. A recent account covers his work on these problems.

B. F. Skinner is, of course, extremely important for much of the research reported in many chapters to follow. In 1959 he published a personal account of the development of his research approach. In his college days, although he had no courses in psychology, he had read about John B. Watson and studied Loeb and Pavlov. In his book he recounted these readings briefly, and next reported that he was at Harvard as a graduate student. It is plausible to infer, from this, that these men most influenced Skinner to follow a career in psychology. In another book, which mentions remarkably few psychologists by name, Skinner refers only to Darwin, Freud, Pavlov, and Thorndike more than twice. All four men were cast in historical perspective and as initiating major developments in psychology. His dependence upon the work of Pavlov may be inferred from his early work, The Behavior of Organisms. By 1938 he had some conception of his research plans for the future but had had only a few years to carry them out. As a consequence he had to depend upon the work of other men in his presentation. It would be no great exaggeration to say that in this work he referred to Pavlov as often as all other men combined.

Nevertheless, Skinner insists that the physiological activity which Pavlov thought he was studying was inferential. The processes being studied by Pavlov had not been reduced to neural events. No direct observations of the cortex are reported. In his view, Pavlov's achievement consisted, not in describing neural processes, but in formulating quantitative relations in behavior. It was in espousing the study of the behavior of the empty organism that he parted company with Pavlov. In short, it is unnecessary to concern oneself with physiological data in order to understand psychological phenomena. As Greenspoon put it, in introducing his chapter on verbal conditioning, Skinner made it possible to see verbal behavior as a response in its own right. Hefferline, in his statement of learning theory, speaks of work in the area less clogged with surplus meaning. Nevertheless, it should be noted in passing that this attempt to eliminate "physiologizing" has been criticized sharply by Pratt, Kohler and Hebb. The chapters in the section in this volume on psychophysiology show that there is still vigor to this approach. Moreover, the chapter by Hefferline attempts to demonstrate that Skinner's general approach is not vitiated by dealing with the internal environment.

It would appear that Pavlov's influence on relatively recent work in learning has been sufficiently demonstrated, but Darwin's more general influence has been neglected to this point. Before closing this discussion of learning some comment seems indicated. As to the implications for later chapters of the work stimulated by Darwin, it is perhaps directly most pertinent to Levine's chapter on the effects of early experience upon adult behavior and to Wolpe's chapter on experimental approaches to neuroses. What began with the work following Darwin in the study of the continuity of mind in animals and man has reached such a degree of acceptance that these chapters are written without any except incidental reference to human subjects. Presumably only poorly controlled research exists with our species. Moreover, the feasibility of using much more radical experimental conditions than would be possible with humans is a compelling reason for the use of lower animals.

In his chapter Levine states that recent interest in his topic comes from Hebb 's emphasis upon perceptual learning and the observations of European ethologists on early social stimulation and its later effect on various species of birds. This historical introduction should be significant to the clinician, who is apt to interpret present research in the perspective of his own interests. Hearing of the work on the effect of deprivation of animals and lacking historical information, the clinician might plausibly assume that the historical sequence was from Freud's theory of psychosexual stages to the work of Spitz, and thence to the animal work. He would thus be misled by what he thinks should have happened. The work on animal deprivation does indeed have clinical implications, but its historical roots are elsewhere. If the clinician does not appreciate the possibility that a problem with clinical significance may have a non clinical origin, he would find much current work difficult to comprehend.

Communication

The chapter on small group research, by Petrullo, best illustrates the relation of communication research to clinical psychology. Clearly, in this area we are dealing simultaneously with a limited aspect of social psychology and with a special problem in learning. It is the social psychological aspect that will be stressed.

Murphy, Murphy and Newcomb state that the first systematic studies of suggestion performed by Braid between 1841 and 1860 represent the inception of experimentation in social psychology. Braid rejected the concept of Mesmerism as magical in nature and invented the term "hypnotism" to describe the experimentally obtained phenomena. At one and the same time there occurred the beginning of experimentation in social psychology and the opening up of experimental research on a clinical problem. Following the work of Braid, there was a long procession of investigations concerned with related phenomena, including those by Ambroise-Auguste Liebeault, Hippolyte Bernheim, Jean Charcot, Pierre Janet, Boris Sidis, and Morton Prince. The work initiated by Bernheim had repercussions in other areas of psychology also. For example, Charcot's pupil, Gustave LeBon, stimulated by his teacher's doctrine of dissociation, found in it the explanation of crowd phenomena as a consequence of the splitting of personality.

A slight trickle of experimental reports concerning group or communication problems appeared throughout the years until World War I. After the war, W. Moede and F. H. Allport independently advanced pleas that social psychology could and should be placed upon an experimental basis. Moede's work, beginning in 1913 with research on co-acting groups (as distinguished from face-to face groups), had priority over that of Allport. Moede studied the introduction of the social variable into standard experiments, such as the threshold of audibility. He did this by comparing the results obtained with subjects working alone with those found when subjects were working in groups of two or more. Using a similar experimental design, he studied imitation, fixation of attention, and learning. His work was not widely known in the United States, partly because the book that gives his major findings was not translated. Munsterberg, at Harvard, being familiar with his results, encouraged F. H. Allport to carry on studies in this area; these launched a whole series of studies.

Face-to-face studies were slower to appear than those on co-acting groups. In connection with priorities in this field, Allport states that the earliest experimental studies were performed by the Russians. They had been stimulated to this work by their concern for individual, as contrasted with collective, behavior-for example, the study of Bechterev and DeLange. These studies, however, did not make much impression upon psychology in the United States.

Lewin 's studies bring us almost to the present. His work, probably arrived at independently of the Russian work, stems directly from Gestalt tradition and to some extent from the work of Moreno. Lewin and his co-workers introduced the concept of social climate or group atmosphere in a research setting. Thereafter this work was to have a pronounced effect on research in social psychology. Variation in productivity of subjects was studied under so-called "authoritarian," "democratic," and "laissez faire" working conditions. Despite the fact that unwarranted generalizations were derived from them, the studies have demonstrated that face-to-face groups could be studied under reasonably well controlled conditions.

Research expanded rapidly after the work of Lewin. Interest in research study spread to community, industrial, and therapeutic research settings. Group dynamics, group cohesion, group decision, and group conflict became intensively studied issues. In 1945 the Massachusetts Institute of Technology Research Center for Group Dynamics was established. In 1948, after the death of Lewin, the Center was moved to the University of Michigan. The Tavistock Institute, located in London, follows in some respects the Lewinian tradition. Under the joint sponsorship of the Center and the Institute a periodical, Human Relations, has appeared which is devoted to research in this area. Deutsch has written a very useful review of Lewin 's work and that inspired by him in the setting of field theory as a way of thinking. These comments about small group research are extended in a later chapter in this volume by Petrullo. Because the "small group" includes within its rubric the face-to-face interaction of two individuals, this historical discussion is also relevant to the chapters by Matarazzo and by Strupp.

Behavior Modification

"Behavior modification," as used as a section heading in this book, covers a multitude of approaches. It includes behavior modification as shown in the structured interview, in verbal conditioning, in the production of experimental neuroses, and in patient-doctor relationships. In a broader sense, the topic of behavior modification is related to the whole field of learning. Studies of behavior modification are studies of learning with a particular intent-the clinical goal of treatment. For example, Wolpe in his consideration of experimental approaches to the neuroses defines them as learned habits acquired in anxiety generating situations. In his chapter he discusses experimental neuroses and behavior therapy, including his own work in psychotherapy through reciprocal inhibition. In his book devoted to the topic Wolpe acknowledged his debt especially to Pavlov and to Hull, although Thorndike, Watson, Tolman, and Skinner are also specifically mentioned. The topic of behavior modification also has a close relation with communication in face-to-face pairs. It is, in fact, correct to say that the psychological study of behavioral modification began with the studies of Bernheim in the middle of the last century. Since his particular technique was that of hypnotic suggestion, a psychotherapeutic technique, his pioneer study is directly relevant.

The study of the behavioral effects of non psychological agents, such as drugs or operations, is an obscure and unwritten phase of the history of psychology. Although it is somewhat more peripheral in nature than the other matters considered here, it is fair to make at least one comment-in this area, the earliest work in the modern tradition was that of Kraepelin.

In a more specific way, recent research on behavioral modification is separable into two phases-the formal and the contentual. This is a distinction that we make in conversational behavior between what is said and how the speaker says it. Formal analysis is concerned with how it is said and includes measurement of speed of talking, length of pauses, rate of talking, expressive movements, gestures, and facial expressions. Although studies of movements, gestures, and facial expressions are not unknown, in later chapters more attention is paid to the temporal relations in speaking.

Studies in the formal phase of behavioral modification were initiated by the work of Chapple, an anthropologist, who published what he called the quantitative analysis of the interaction of individuals. At that time he was concerned neither with the interview nor with behavior modification. He saw the method of study he developed in the broader perspective of methodology for anthropological and social psychological study. Chapple saw as a weakness the fact that with the original primitive apparatus only two individuals could be studied simultaneously. The original studies were designed to give the durations of "actions" and "inactions" for calculation of the cumulative plot and the subsequent study and interpretation of the slope of the curves obtained. Later this interaction method was applied to the interview and behavior modification. By 1946 was referring to the period of time with the subjects as an "interview." This interaction method in the interview forms the basis for the studies reported in a later chapter by Matarazzo. Since this chapter contains a thorough review, attention hereafter will now be directed to the contentual phases of research on behavior modification.

The research study of the contentual phase of behavior modification by psychotherapy is a relatively new development. Its recent appearance cannot be attributed to a lack of an earlier literature on psychotherapy. Psychotherapy had been recognized as a specialized technique at least as early as the temple medicine of the Greeks in about the fifth century before Christ. Its rich history is attested to in various detailed accounts. Nor was an extensive modern professional literature lacking. Individual psychotherapy has been a concern for a large number of clinical workers for a considerable number of years. A vast literature was already developing before 1940. Moreover, psychologists, as distinguished from other clinicians, had been engaging in psychotherapy and recounting their experiences with it since before 1910, as witness the work of Boris Sidis and Walter Dill Scott. Material was available on many issues and problems, even for as specialized a problem as group psychotherapy, for Slavson was able to cite forty articles published from 1905 to 1939. Nevertheless, until quite recently the published work relied on anecdotal methods supplemented by gross statistical findings. In evaluating psychoanalytic therapy as late as 1941, Knight reported an evaluation in which he had to fall back upon brochures of various institutes and a count of the number "cured," "better," and the like for his sources of information. Pleas for a research approach to the contentual phase of behavior modification had been made directly or indirectly in the twenties and thirties by Lasswell, Rosenzweig, Saul and Symonds. In fact, Lasswell went beyond this appeal to report some data on electrically recorded psycho analytic sessions.

It was a psychologist, Carl Rogers, who in 1942, through a book and an article, launched the research approach in behavioral modification through psychotherapy.

Rogers' work needs no review here; we will move, instead, to a brief evaluation of early workers who influenced him. It is fashionable when speaking of Rogers to allege his debt to Otto Rank, to Jessie Taft, and possibly to Frederick Allen. All of these are non psychologists. To my inquiry concerning his indebtedness to psychology, Rogers replied, in a personal communication:

So far as psychology goes, I guess I would say that Goodwin Watson and Leta Hollingworth of Teachers College, Columbia, both had real impact on me. E. K. Wickman of the Institute for Child Guidance was another psychologist whose thinking had some effect on me. Watson was very independent in his thinking and gave his students a great deal of freedom. Leta Hollingworth was an excellent clinician. Wickman was the careful, thoughtful, cautious researcher, though not a research man in a laboratory sense.

These three psychologists shared the tendency, which Rogers attributes to Wickman, to carry their research beyond the laboratory. None of them would be called an experimental psychologist in the narrow sense. Yet all three shared in that laboratory tradition through the training they themselves had received, and all three maintained familiarity with experimental work. It is as if Rogers had grandparents who were from among the experimentalists. Directly relevant to the issue at hand is a thoughtful article by Rogers written to describe the conflict and resulting gap that he felt existed between his work as a psychotherapist and his work as a researcher. His personal reconciliation, recounted therein, is an exercise in the reconciliation of the clinical and experimental traditions.

Rogers' work typifies still another way that the experimental tradition in psychology operates. He brought to the problem of psychotherapy neither a particular approach nor a problem analogous to an early experimental one, but a tendency to transfer his research training. He and his students, challenged by the problem of quantification of the process of psychotherapy, used ingeniously a variety of psychological tools-recording devices, rating scales, and so on-to attack the problem. They approached it with an internalized experimental tradition and, basing their methods on this tradition, proceeded to work with the materials of clinical psychology.

Rogers' influence upon his own students and others is direct and obvious in many instances. It probably influenced many other psychologists who by no stretch of the imagination could be called "Rogerian." Many research studies bearing no direct obligation to his particular work but stimulated by it, came about once it was realized that Rogers had made a "breakthrough" in this area of research, although these studies were quite different in nature.

2

Experimental Bases of Personality Assessment

Introduction

Early in the nineteenth century the German philosopher and psychologist Johann Herbart wrote that psychology was a science- and a mathematical science. He said, furthermore, that psychology was empirical but could not be experimental, for, as Boring remarked, Herbart saw no way in which experimentation could be done on the mind. Herbart was wrong, but by denying that psychology could be an experimental science he issued a challenge that stimulated scholars to attack the problem. A major breakthrough came in the form of the Weber-Fechner law, which showed that at least one aspect of mental phenomena-sensation-could be studied by means of physical responses to known stimuli. Although the law had only limited application, it pointed the way to other experimental investigations of behavior, which eventually included personality measurement.

The new interest in research on behavior led, of course, to blind alleys and false starts-for example, Lombroso 's notion that criminality was inborn and that the criminal type could be identified by means of measurable and classifiable physical stigmata; or the theory advanced by Gall, a Viennese anatomist, that personality and other traits were reflected by bumps and other irregularities on the surface of the skull. These early (nineteenth-century) attempts to relate physical structure to personality were quickly rejected as pseudoscientific, although echoes of the theories linger on in the folkways.

Unfortunately, a by-product of the disillusionment with such theories seems to be a general indifference to and contempt for subsequent attempts in the twentieth century which were genuinely scientific. In particular, Kretschmer's work on constitutional psychology, initiated after World War I and greatly extended in recent decades by Sheldon, merits serious consideration. Hall and Lindzey have an excellent discussion of work in this area.

But if there were blind alleys in the scientific study of behavior, there were also rich and rewarding leads. In the 1880's, as cases in point, Sir Francis Galton, ably followed by James McKeen Cattell, measured individual differences and devised some early statistical techniques for analyzing them. Out of this work came the first psychological tests in the modem tradition. At turn of the present century, Binet and Simon, taking another long step forward, developed the intelligence test. Their unique contribution probably lies in their concept of mental age as a basis for scaling intellectual performance. Significantly, current practice in intelligence assessment still utilizes their ideas. The remaining names and techniques which should be mentioned are relatively recent. The major contributors include E. L. Thorndike, R. S. Woodworth, L. M. Terman, Cyril Burt, L. L. Thurstone, Hermann Rorschach; the instruments developed include the Vocational Interest Blank, Murray's Thematic Apperception Test (TAT), Wechsler's intelligence scales, Kuder's Preference Record, Kent-Rosanoff Word Association Test, and Hathaway's Minnesota Multiphasic Personality Inventory (MMPI).

With this brief historical background in mind, we may go on to review present-day attempts to measure personality and personality change. The approaches differ widely and the evidence gathered varies in quality, but all are concerned with obtaining valid answers to crucial questions. There are a number of ways in which the many methods of personality assessment might be classified. The categories used here are modifications of those used by Berg in a review article.

Because of the present stage of personality assessment research, a good many of the studies reviewed in following pages are not fully experimental, even within a charitable interpretation of the term. But because they are pertinent, we must include them if we are to understand the scope of assessment research today.

Rating Methods

In assessing personality the most frequently used method is that of rating. Particular rating techniques vary immensely in form and content. They may be short and simple checklists or lengthily elegant scales. Usually they call for written responses such as words or check marks, but upon occasion the responses may be oral, gestural, or something else. The setting may require an immediate rating, as is the case during interviews or sociometric observations. At other times, a leisured recollection of past incidents may be required prior to rating. But in every instance one person judges another. He may pool his ratings with others and he may rate persons in a group; yet the basis of rating remains typically individual and subjective. The factor of subjectivity has justly troubled many researchers, because ratings in general have rather low reliability and their validity is difficult to establish. Yet in most clinical situations no other method is feasible. Despite their weaknesses, rating methods are convenient and often provide a useful comprehensive estimate of personality. In any case, whatever the yearnings of a scientifically oriented clinician may be, there is really no escaping ratings. More than one veteran researcher has smiled sourly when urged by a neophyte to use the MMPI or similar instrument as an objective personality measure in order to avoid ratings. The veteran knows that the MMPI is an excellent test, but he also knows that ratings were originally involved in identifying the MMPI criterion groups and in the subjects' self-ratings when responding to the test items, as well as in the interpretation of the scores. Ratings are indeed always with us; and our task becomes one of understanding and improving, not of decrying them.

Actually, rating techniques have a quite respectable scientific ancestry in classical psychophysics; the problems lie in how to use them neatly, with a maximum of rigor. As Stevens has noted, both psychological tests and rating methods may be viewed as psycho physical procedures. With this in mind, we may review the categories of persons who do the ratings and then examine the factors which, at times, lead them astray. Raters may be placed in one of three categories: professional, such as the staff members of a hospital; self, where the subject or patient evaluates himself; others, such as the family, friends, or co-workers of the subject.

Professional Ratings

Professional raters are those who have some special competence in the behavioral area under investigation. Nurses and hospital aides, for example, usually have the most accurate information concerning a patient's daily ward behavior, while the social worker is often best able to rate the patient's relationship to his family. Behavioral dynamics or specific diagnostic judgments are best appraised by psychologists or psychiatrists. The most reliable ratings come about when the professional rates in the area for which his training and experience have best equipped him. Ratings from various sources are often pooled in order to increase reliability and validity. In clinic staff meetings for example, individual clinical ratings are reviewed collectively; in experimental studies summed ratings are employed in order to define or identify some variable.

Self-ratings

Personality and adjustment may be affected by psychotherapy or by disease or injury. The technique most commonly employed for finding evidence of such personality modification is patient self-ratings, which are secured in a variety of ways. The crudest, most informal form would be an instance in which the patient's volunteered remark-"I feel better/worse today"-is woven into the fabric of someone else's rating. Still informal, but more deliberate, would be the probe in the form of the fatuous question, "How are we today?" But self-ratings typically involve more formal techniques, including perhaps oral reports derived from lengthy interviews and detailed rating forms; sometimes the ratings are obtained in before-, during-, and after-treatment appraisals, a desirable technique.

The value of many kinds of self-reports is reduced, however, by the influence of powerful cultural factors. For example, when asked, "How do you feel?" the out-patient who is still inter-acting socially in the outside world may respond, "Much better, thanks," simply because the acquiescent response is the rule in our society. Hathaway has discussed this response characteristic at some length as the "Hello Goodbye" pattern. Or another factor may operate in this sort of situation: since no one enjoys being regarded as a fool, the patient may be unwilling to suggest that his and the therapist's time have been utterly wasted, and so claim a change for the better no matter how he really feels.

Opposed to this broad cultural set for acquiescence is the specific reinforcement of "sick" responses, particularly among hospitalized patients. The patient who says he feels fine get little attention from the ward nurse or aide; the patient who mentions a Martian on his back or a bomb in his belly gets attention from the aide, the nurse, the ward physician, and perhaps even a consultant. It seems obvious therefore that the patient's self-ratings are unlikely to reflect personality changes with any validity.

Ratings by Others

Occasionally a patient's family and/or others who know him have been asked to rate him on various personality dimensions. Because such ratings may be a source of embarrassment to the patient or to the person doing the rating, they are not usually trustworthy. Furthermore, the raters may ardently desire to have the patient back home or at work or, with equal ardor, want him kept in the hospital. Such emotional involvement is more the rule than the exception among a patient's family and friends. Thus, these ratings are of little value for the experimental study of personality, unless the study is directed at the raters rather than the patients who are being rated.

The reliability and validity of ratings: In our discussion thus far, ratings have been described as having serious weaknesses. Yet-to repeat an earlier point-we cannot really avoid them in personality assessment. Fortunately, ratings can be reliable and valid, particularly when done by professionals under carefully structured conditions. The Hospital Adjustment Scale (HAS) by McReynolds, Ballachey and Ferguson, for example, can be filled out by a nurse or aide in about ten minutes; yet its reliability is reasonably high, as is the Multidimensional Scale for Rating Psychiatric Patients (MSRPP) by Lorr, Singer, and Zobel designed for use by psychologists and psychiatrists. The two scales were compared by Stilson, Mason, Gynther and Gertz in a study which required student nurses to rate 36 neuropsychiatric patients on the HAS while psychologists rated the same patients on the MSRPP. When the patients were re-rated by the same groups, the HAS had a reliability of .79; the MSRPP, of .80. The correlation between HAS and MSRPP ratings was - .57, indicating not only a satisfactory level of reliability for the individual scales but also reasonable agreement between the two sets of raters. It also appears that when the task is properly structured for them, student nurses can do a competent job of rating neuropsychiatric patients. Lorr, one of the authors of the MSRPP, has a comprehensive survey of rating scales which will be useful to those contemplating research that involves these methods.

Even self-ratings can be reliable under certain conditions. Webb reported that the reliability of self-ratings vs. re-ratings for normal subjects was only .19 when they were asked to give a quantitative rating of themselves along a single dimension. However, when he had the subjects compare themselves with other members of the group, he found that the reliability of their ratings was now at the respectable range of .58 to .91, despite the fact that self-ratings were used. Of course, subjects with severe emotional disturbances would probably be less consistent in self-ratings.

Although professional personnel, by and large, do a better job of rating, in terms of reliability and validity, than do other groups, even professional ratings cannot always be trusted. In the hospital situation, for example, the wise, experimentally oriented clinician is wary of ratings of patient improvement as reflected in rates of patients discharged. This is particularly true of crowded state hospitals, where the rate of patients discharged as improved increases with increased pressure for new admissions. Occasionally a carefully designed research has failed simply because its success depended upon a professional rating which turned out to be slovenly. Schofield's carefully executed attempt to construct a "susceptibility to therapy" scale for the MMPI failed because patients in his criterion group were discharged from the hospital as improved when actually they were not.

But the pitfalls of rating techniques can be avoided and ratings can often make a surprisingly good showing. Intelligence measurement, for example, is often regarded as the unique province for particular tests. However, Hanna found that ratings of intelligence based upon material from carefully conducted interviews correlated .71 with the American Council on Education Psychological Examination and .66 with the Ohio State University Psychological Test. The two tests correlated .77 with each other; hence the intelligence estimate based upon ratings appears to be virtually as good as either test. Similar validity evidence for ratings is reflected in Wittson and Hunt's examination of 944 Navy neuropsychiatric (NP) discharges in relation to ratings by psychiatrists and psychologists as to degree of NP disability. Of those servicemen rated mild disability, only 6.5 per cent were later discharged as NP cases; of those rated moderate, 20.2 per cent were eventually NP discharges; but 89.7 per cent of those rated severe were later discharged for NP conditions. This study is a good example of how ratings may be effectively employed to achieve satisfactory validity and reliability, for the raters were professionally trained in the area they were rating, and no fine discriminations were demanded. Had they been required to rate severity of NP disability on a 20-point scale, the results would probably not have been so impressive. Indeed, Hunt, Wittson, and Hunt did something along these lines when they studied specificity of diagnostic rating and percentage of agreement among raters at a Navy pre commissioning station and at a hospital. The subjects rated were 794 naval enlisted men. There was 93.7 per cent agreement for the rating "unsuitable for service"; however with somewhat greater rating specificity, the percentage of agreement was 54.1 for such categories as "psychosis," "psychoneurosis." When particular disorders were listed, such as "schizophrenia," "hysteria," or "anxiety state," the percentage of agreement was 32.6. If further specificity had been sought (for example, categories of paranoid schizophrenia), the level of agreement would undoubtedly have dropped even further.

It seems clear that ratings may or may not be useful, depending upon who does them, and how. At this point it is worth while to examine the conditions under which useful, reliable, and valid ratings may be obtained. Those researchers who successfully employ rating methods have observed a few simple precautions. A fairly short distillation of the necessary guide lines, such as those suggested by Pinillos, should be all that is needed for experimental-clinical purposes.

Careful selection of raters is essential. The rater must have competence in the area he is appraising. Curiously, nearly everyone considers himself to be an expert in the assessment of behavior. Beyond competence there are characteristics associated with good raters. Good judges tend to be task-oriented and socially detached, as Taft emphasized, whereas poor raters are less stable and introceptive. Thus the good rater in appraising sociability might give weight to the subject's having been elected to office in a civic club, while the poor rater might be strongly influenced by his friendly smile. In other words, poor raters are more likely to generalize and exhibit the halo effect. Other factors also contribute to poor ratings. For example, Taft has remarked that members of minority groups and rural dwellers do not rate well, although the reasons for this are not clear. Similarly, other characteristics of raters or rates can affect the kind of appraisal made. Intelligence and education, according to Bendig can influence ratings. So can the particular situation, as in Landfield 's finding that subjects predicted their own behavior less accurately when in the presence of threatening persons than they did in the presence of non threatening persons. Rankin and Campbell found that white subjects exhibit a greater magnitude of galvanic skin response to Negro than to white examiners. Presumably, ratings taken under any of these conditions would be directly affected by the conditions. However, such findings do not negate the use of ratings; rather, they underline the importance of selecting raters carefully.

It is essential that the rater have time and opportunity to observe the rate. As crucial as careful selection of raters is the additional condition that the raters know the pertinent behavior of the person being rated. More than one investigator has ignored this point while clearly defining the rater's qualifications in terms of training and experience. Occasionally this omission comes painfully to light only when an earnest rater writes on his form, "I think the patient is better, but I saw him only once for five minutes about a month ago." When such omissions do not come to light, the ratings may simply be condemned as useless and the study abandoned. Or worse-the study is published as a melange of inconsistencies, to provide fresh ammunition for the non clinical psychologists who gleefully collect examples of clinical nonsense mislabeled "research." Holzberg has stressed the importance of accumulating pertinent information before attempting to rate, but this sound injunction is often ignored on the dangerous assumption that a rater will not rate a person when he knows little or nothing about him. Some raters won't, of course, but some will and do. The only safeguards are to make certain that each rater understands the basis of personal knowledge upon which he is to make his judgment, and to make provision on the rating form for indications of the kind of information upon which the rating is based.

It is essential that rater bias be eliminated or controlled. This has already been mentioned in passing references to such factors as the "halo" effect wherein a favorable or unfavorable trait colors the rater's judgment of all other traits. But there are many other forms of bias: Specialized experiences or particular responsibilities, for example, may produce emotional identifications which interfere with valid ratings. Understandably, therefore, American scientists who are developing space missiles will rate our achievements ahead of the Russians, while the generals in charge of United States defense programs rate us lagging behind; or most American physicians may rate American medicine as the "best in the world," and our professional educators appraise American education in identical superlatives. The same physicians can usually validly and reliably assess the efficacy of one drug over another in treating a particular disease, and the same educators can often decide with reasonable objectivity that one method of teaching arithmetic is better than another. The latter ratings are in the area of their professional competence and, with a well-defined rating task, can be relatively free from bias. But being a member of a profession, like being a member of a family, has powerful emotional involvements, and it is too much to expect objectivity where emotional identification is primary. The possibility of such biases must be explored, and the biases controlled. Should bias exist, it does not mean that a rating cannot be made. The quality of American medicine could perhaps be appraised by members of kindred, but non-M.D., professions or another national group. For example, Swiss physicians might rate a large number of specific features on a paired-comparison basis in which first British and American, then French and American medicine were compared. Certain objective factors might also be included for assessment, such as death rate, epidemics, stillbirths. Thus, rater bias may be controlled or eliminated to a considerable extent, but one must first pinpoint it.

It is essential that the characteristics to be rated be expressed in simple, objective, and well-defined form. Bias is not the only source of possible distortion in ratings; They may also be distorted simply because the rater does not know what he is supposed to rate. Worse, he may think he knows when actually something else is desired. Candidates for executive positions have frequently been rated on such characteristics as trustworthiness, future promise, stability; but unless such items are cast in behavioral and situational terms the ratings are likely to be meaningless. Thus trustworthiness can mean discharging all responsibilities on schedule, or accuracy and honesty in handling money. Which is to be rated? In the same way, future promise may be appraised only in situational terms-future promise for what? An engineer may be quite ordinary as an engineer but bear bright promise as an executive vice-president. Similarly, stability in bank presidents may be quite different from stability in sales managers. Such terms are obviously deceptive and require definition. To avoid misunderstanding, a description of the duties involved in the new situation should be spelled out before asking for ratings. For example, "This position is research director of an NP 2000 bed private hospital. The director supervises and coordinates the work of four assistant directors who are Ph.D.'s in psychology, and he deals directly with consultants in psychiatry, social work, anthropology, and statistics. He must be experienced in the design and appraisal of research with neuropsychiatric patients, particularly the treatment of schizophrenics and alcoholics. It is very important that he be able to present clear reports, both oral and written, to professional and lay groups, etc." The idea is to give details of the situation and the responsibilities of the job. Then, if the rater knows the person he is rating, he can do a much better job in his appraisal. He can even determine when he must say, "I don't know how he would perform in such a situation."

Occasionally, a rating form is over elaborate, and in this case, too, its purpose may be defeated. As Sorenson and Gross noted, complex rating forms often cause confusion. The confused rater does a poor rating job; the irritated rater usually abandons the task in frustration. Careful pilot testing will provide the means for identifying and correcting such sources of error.

There is, then, no escape from ratings. The experimental clinician would do well to recognize the usefulness of rating procedures for appraising any facet of personality and personality change. Ratings can be reliable and valid when biases are identified, controlled, or eliminated; rating scales can be confusing, but they need not be, for good scales can be prepared, often with less trouble than poor scales. The investigator in personality research must at some point deal with data obtained by rating methods; he may as well learn to use them effectively.

Psychological Test Methods

In a review which may be recommended to any serious student of the problem at hand, Super observed that fads and fancies appear in theories and techniques of personality assessment. Once the professional psychology journals were full of articles dealing with measures of ascendance-submission, expressive-movement, introversion-extroversion, but now such studies are rare. After a decade of virtual oblivion, a few studies of expressive movement have recently begun to reappear. During the past half-dozen years, Super notes, interest has waxed and then waned in research on personality characteristics such as authoritarianism, rigidity, empathy, motivation, and anxiety. A rash of studies has appeared in the past on each of these topics, followed by a gradual drop-off in frequency, as indicated by publication in Psychological Abstracts or The Annual Review of Psychology. Certain instruments, however, seem to endure the pounding of each newest tool, outlasting the fad as the anvil outlasts the hammer. The Minnesota Multiphasic Personality Inventory (MMPI), for example, has gained steadily in usefulness and clinical importance over the years. This is not too surprising in view of the amazing flexibility of this test. If social introversion is in the air, professionally speaking, or configural scoring of tests, Drake has a scale for the former and Meehl a method for the latter. One would be hard put to think of a new fad which the MMPI could not exploit by means of a new scale or new technique.

Projective Techniques

In view of the firm foundation of supporting empirical evidence, it is not surprising that the MMPI has proved durable and useful; it is surprising that the Rorschach is still in the clinical armamentorium. Kelly wondered whether the adherence to such tests as the Rorschach, in view of the absence of demonstrated predictive validity, was not a phenomenon that should be studied by social psychologists. Super (1959) has observed that Eysenck reported abandoning the Rorschach as a clinical tool at the Maudsley Hospital in England, but that Columbia University continues to require a large block of graduate student time dedicated to projective techniques, despite dissatisfaction with them. In Super's words:

> We have agreed that they have no validity, but we retain the requirement. We do this for three reasons: (1) The unsatisfactory but practical consideration that such psychologists are expected to have these skills and are likely to both feel and be handicapped if they do not, (2) the fact that they can learn something useful about clinical interaction by studying these procedures, and (3) the hope that familiarity with these methods may yet provide psychologists with a basis for some major breakthrough in the field of personality assessment.

It seems probable that Super's candid statement would be echoed by the staff members in many other clinical psychology programs where the research literature on projective techniques is known. Unquestionably, the validity of the Rorschach is very low, however, a new approach may emerge which will preserve the attractive, perceptual features of the Rorschach and still yield solid evidence for predictive validity. Perhaps the objective scoring approach of Holtzman or the stimulus analysis research by Baughman will provide the key. For the experimental clinician, the Annual Review of Psychology offers a year-by-year account of the status of research on the Rorschach and other projective techniques, as well as on new and provocative lines of inquiry.

Objective Personality Inventories

The adjective objective as applied to personality appraisal can be something of a problem. For present purposes, however, objectivity in personality measures may be considered achieved when the scoring of test responses by different persons shows little variance. As noted in the section on Rating Methods, the interpretation of such objectively determined scores may still be subjective, even though the scores are not. Three procedures have generally been followed in developing objective measures of personality. Edwards has described them as: (1) factor analysis techniques, (2) the criterion group method, (3) construct approaches.

Factor analysis technique has been used by Guilford in his Inventory of Factors STDCR and by Cattell in the 16 PF Questionnaire. The basic assumption of this approach is that a small number of factors will emerge from a large number of items. Just what these factors will be is not known in advance; hence close scrutiny of the content of those items which have high loadings for a particular factor is necessary. From such examination it is possible to get a more or less definite idea of what the items have in common. Then a label is applied which seems to be reasonably descriptive of the factor. It is at this point that difficulty is encountered, at least from the standpoint of clinical practice. A factor designated as sociability may mean various things to various clinicians, ranging from the overt manifestations of sociability exhibited by the backslapping politician to an undemonstrative but sincere enjoyment of just being with other people. A further description of the factor is usually supplied in order to clarify the term; however, the confusion is not necessarily dispelled, perhaps because the label, not the extended description, is what sticks in the mind of the clinician. As a result, some writers have used letters or numbers for their factors and then offered an explanation in terms of the content of the items which make up the factor. Cattell has frequently done this and given a description of negative and positive loadings, such as "impulsive, generous versus close, cautious." He also makes up words like premsia, alaxia, or parmia, apparently on the assumption that old associations will be less likely to be present in the new word. Whatever the drawbacks, factor methods do provide a means for scaling a single personality variable.

The criterion group method, called the "group difference method" by Super, requires two groups defined on some reasonably operational basis. The Strong Vocational Interest Blank, for example, used "men in general" for one group, and "engineers" for the other in preparing one of the occupational keys. The MMPI similarly employed a group of normal persons and a group of schizophrenics in the preparation of the Sc scale. With this method, after the groups have been appropriately identified, both are given a set of stimulus material, such as test items, and the responses are recorded. Those responses which differentiate the two groups at some agreed-upon level of statistical significance are then used as the basis for constructing a scale. This provides a straightforward empirical method of selecting items for measuring the variable under study. There are advantages and disadvantages to this approach. The experimenter has a scale based upon the responses of groups of known characteristics; thus when using the scale, he can predict with reasonable accuracy whether the scores indicate that a given subject responds like the members of one group or the other. The accuracy of this prediction, however, is limited to the representativeness of the groups originally used. This can be a problem, for contamination does occur despite careful application of controls. A large group of normal subjects, for example, is likely to include some persons who are "normal" only in the sense of not being hospitalized. Conversely, a group of schizophrenics will sometimes include patients who are really no longer schizophrenic but who, for various reasons, continue to be tagged with this NP classification. Another aspect of the problem of identifying criterion groups resides in locating meaningful operational definitions. Maturity in the sense of chronological age, for example, can be satisfactorily defined from birth certificates; however, something like delinquency is not amenable to convenient definition. Some who are called delinquents are merely neglected children, while others are schizophrenics, psychopaths, etc. Further information on the problem of criterion group definition will be found in Edwards' and Berg's discussions.

When using the construct approach, the investigator has a fairly definite idea of some variable that he wishes to study. He then devises items which are intended to sample its behavioral facets. Thus, if he is interested in behavior relating to religion, he may prepare items which deal with attendance at church, frequency of prayer, etc., and which are intended to tap aspects of a construct which might be termed, after Allport, Vernon, and Lindzey, religious values or perhaps religiosity. The items thus obtained are administered to a heterogeneous group of subjects and the responses are analyzed, usually by factorial methods, in order to identify those items which relate most closely to each other and thus appear to be related to the construct. From such items a scale may then be prepared. Several tests, such as the Study of Values and the Personal Preference Schedule were developed in this way.

The construct method has an advantage in that the investigator knows what he has striven to put into his items from the very beginning and he can employ factor analytical or other techniques to appraise the relation of particular items to the construct. Also, as Edwards has observed, this is a form of the criterion group approach, with the important difference that item responses, not external criteria, identify the groups. Edwards goes on to note that different investigators may map a construct differently with the result that, while both use the same labels, the scales developed by each may be different. The same difficulty is reflected in the initial preparation of items. If an important area of the construct remains untapped, the scale will be inadequate. Factor analysis techniques have the advantage with regard to this point, for the large, commonly employed pool of heterogeneous items is much more likely to sample a broad range of behavior than the restricted content of items used in the construct approach. For such broader sampling, one pays a price in the form of an unwieldy factor matrix. But when it comes to labeling the variable, the construct method offers an advantage in that one may reasonably assume that what was put into the items should come out in the scale. It may be noted that neither statistical treatment nor labels are a problem in the criterion group approach if the groups are validly defined.

It is not feasible to examine in detail the many research and clinical uses of psychological tests, for the number of articles published is staggering. During the 20 years the MMPI has been in existence approximately a thousand studies dealing with the single test have appeared in print. The Rorschach is a considerably older test; hence it may not be surprising to learn that more than three thousand articles on it have been published. These are but two tests; and while they are among the most popular of all personality tests, there are hundreds of others about which many articles have been published. In clinical experimentation the tests are commonly used under test-retest conditions. That is, the test is given prior to the introduction of some new condition, such as therapeutic treatment, and then administered one or more times afterward. The usual pattern is testing once before and once after therapy. Rarely does a given study report follow-up testing after the formal therapeutic effort has been terminated.

The assumption underlying this test-retest procedure is that the tests will adequately measure the disturbed personality state prior to treatment, and the retest will reflect any personality changes which result from the treatment. Both assumptions are questionable. Even the best personality tests have a high percentage of false negative and false positive identifications. The researcher may work with a group of known adjustment characteristics-for example, in a group of schizophrenics; yet the test data will not identify all members of the group as schizophrenics. Furthermore, in the case of diagnostic categories, test score changes do not necessarily mean changes in the severity of the disorder. Thus, while schizophrenics usually earn standard scores above 70 on the MMPI Sc (Schizophrenia) scale, mild cases of schizophrenia may have very low or very high Sc scores, in the neighborhood of 73 or 93, because tests are rarely validated for severity levels in such situations. It is in fact difficult to establish reliably and validly the degrees of severity in psychopathological states, which brings into question the assumption that the test will adequately measure the disturbed behavioral state under investigation. Perhaps a fair appraisal would be to state that present tests identify behavior atypicalities, but not very well.

Even more troublesome is the assumption that test score changes will reflect personality changes, because again tests are not validated for personality changes resulting from intervention such as psychotherapy. Clearly, test scores can change as a function of psychotherapy, but we to date have no methods to find confirming evidence. Thus, when Muench administered several tests to a group of patients before and after psychotherapy, it was not clear whether the tests or the therapy were being validated. If one had good evidence that psychotherapy was successful, then the tests could be validated; conversely, the psychotherapy could be validated for efficacy if it were established that the test scores really changed with effective therapy- and we can recall here the failure of Schofield's research, which stumbled over that very point. Changes in test scores, incidentally, do occur in a test-retest situation; yet they may have nothing whatsoever to do with personality changes. A common phenomenon is regression toward the mean; hence with repeated testing, scores often increase or decrease depending upon whether they were originally below or above the mean. An elementary precaution against such problems is the use of control groups-an obvious safeguard which is lacking in a number of studies. One might also observe that virtually all research on personality change provides no control for the mere passage of time. Disturbed people do sometimes recover without therapy; thus a non treatment control group is essential.

Another problem is that personality tests touch only a small sample of behavior; the range of behavior sampled may be too narrow to reflect adequately whatever changes do occur. Similarly, a particular personality dimension may be measured reasonably well in the normal person-but does it apply to psychopathological states? Is a sociability scale developed for normal persons meaningful when applied to schizophrenics ? It may be, but we do not know that it is. There are many such problems, and they can be answered. But we do not have the answers yet. Perhaps the excitement for experimentally oriented clinicians in behavioral research lies precisely in these unanswered questions.

In summary, then-although personality tests have serious limitations, they are nevertheless useful for the clinician and the researcher so long as they are correctly applied and adequately understood-in terms of both what they can do and how they do it.

Verbal Behavior

The relationship between speech and personality has long been recognized as close; however, most attention in this area of behavior has been directed to what is said or written, rather than to how. As Sanford put it, "Language, traditionally, has been regarded as the 'vehicle of thought,' with the thought attracting far more attention than the vehicle." Jackson and Messick have more recently discussed content and style in relation to personality. The clinician notes the agreement between style and content when a patient slowly and laboriously utters, "I feel depressed, just no good-useless to the world," etc. But our professional habits are such that we typically are more closely attuned to what is said than to other language characteristics.

An example from Berg is to the point:

> *Let us suppose that a client were to say, "I wanted to see you because I know that my boss has it in for me. I know he hates me because of the things he does to me. Even my fellow workers say that my troubles on the job are not what I do but rather what the boss does to me. I won't tell you what I think of him but just let me describe what I've had happen to me at work."*

The alert therapist would undoubtedly recognize the paranoid flavor of this patient's remarks-to the ideational content-but would he also be aware that 15 of the 75 words, or 20 per cent in our sample, were the ego words I, me, and my? The chances are good that the therapist would not have noticed this language characteristic; for his training inclines him toward noticing the ideas expressed rather than the choice of words. Clinically speaking, this is probably sensible in a practical setting; for bizarre notions, thought fragmentation, delusions, etc., are readily apparent in the ideas conveyed by a patient and pertinent to clinical decisions. But for experimental purposes, other language characteristics can be a rich, if little-worked, mine of data for assessing personality and personality change. One of the early studies of this sort in which actual data were gathered was that of Buseman, who found that an increase in verbs as related to adjectives among a group of school children was associated with teachers' ratings of instability among those pupils. Balken and Masserman employed the same verb-adjective ratio in an investigation of the language of 50 patients diagnosed as cases of conversion hysteria, anxiety state, and obsessive-compulsive reaction. They reported that adjectives were used more frequently by the conversion hysterics, while the obsessive compulsive patients used more verbs and more total words. The anxiety-state patients used relatively fewer adjectives and were in between the other groups in frequency of verb usage. A somewhat more carefully executed study is that by Lorenz and Cobb, who compared the spontaneous speech which accompanied TAT testing for 10 hysteric patients with that of 10 control subjects. When compared to the normal group, the hysteric patients were found to use more verbs and pronouns, fewer adjectives, prepositions, conjunctions, and articles. The patients also used the pronoun I with high frequency and used fewer different kinds of words per thousand words uttered. Another study by Lorenz and Cobb reported differences between speech samples of 10 manic and 10 control patients. The manics, like hysterics, used fewer different kinds of words and they repeated particular words with greater than normal frequency. They also used more pronouns, more main and auxiliary verbs, and fewer adjectives and prepositions. In general, the manic speech appeared to be relatively repetitive and homogeneous, unlike normal speech, which qualifies and individualizes.

Again many such studies unfortunately lack appropriate control groups for comparison purposes-for example, a number of language studies of the type-token ratio. These studies have compared the number of different words (the types) with the total number of all words spoken (the tokens) and there is probably something basic and potentially meaningful in such analyses of verbal behavior. Some of the results obtained thus far are tantalizing, although not yet convincing. Mann has shown that normal subjects have a higher type-token ratio (TTR) than schizophrenic patients, and Fairbanks has offered some support in his finding that schizophrenics use significantly fewer nouns, conjunctions, prepositions, and articles, but significantly more verbs, pronouns, and interjections than college students. Roshal used the TTR for the first and last of a series of psychotherapeutic interviews and found changes indicating that increased variability in verbal behavior had occurred, presumably as a result of the treatment. The majority of TTR researches have used college students as subjects or in control groups; and since speech is the response measure employed, it is difficult to assess the possible influence of vocabulary size, verbal fluency, education, etc. The possible existence of such influences does not, however, negate the usefulness of verbal behavioral measures. Speech is, after all, exclusively human and thus may well be a most fertile field for clinical research; but speech is so sensitive to cultural influences of class, education, and intelligence that such research requires controls which are considerably more thoroughgoing than usual.

Other approaches have examined verbal behavior in different contexts and with varying degrees of success. Dollard and Mowrer developed a discomfort-relief quotient (DRQ) to measure behavioral change. This method classifies words, clauses, and sentences as to whether they signify discomfort, relief from discomfort, or neither. Hunt carefully applied the DRQ to social casework settings and found that the ratings of improvement made by case workers failed to correlate significantly with the DRQ. An analysis of broader ideational units expressed by clients during therapeutic interviews was employed by Snyder, who found that the client's discussion of future plans was virtually nonexistent during the first interview, but increased to approximately 12 per cent of the responses in the last interview. He also reported that the affective tone of responses changed from negative to positive during the same period. Seeman in a somewhat similar study also found an increase in positive and a decrease in negative attitudes as therapy progressed. Interestingly, however, he observed that positive attitudes tended to be expressed in the past tense and negative attitudes in the present.

While their method was rather qualitative, Mayers and Mayers did a novel study of the responses of various types of patients who were asked to make up stories. They assumed that the patients' conflicts would be reflected in their syntax and grammatical expression, and found some support for this notion in that insecure individuals used "might" and "if" frequently, whereas passive individuals avoided active verbs in favor of participles and passive expressions. Schizophrenics showed some tendency to omit articles and pronouns. Using a case published by Carl Rogers as his source of data, Berg analyzed a series of eight therapeutic interviews in terms of frequency of ego words (I, me, my, mine, etc.), empathic words (you, we, our, us, etc.), negative expressions (no, never, not, etc.), and the ratio of syllables to words. On the assumption that certain initial word sounds would be associated with profanity and obscenity, he then tabulated the number of words beginning with B, K, F, P, S, and Sh. It was found that, as the interviews progressed, the frequency of ego words decreased and empathic words increased. The frequency of B, K, F, etc., words also decreased with succeeding interviews. The correction of ego word frequency with this word analysis was .80. The negative word frequency showed a decrease as adjustment improved, and the word-syllable ratio showed no significant relationship to any of the measures taken.

Still another technique was that used by Chodorkoff and Mussen in a study of 40 schizophrenic patients compared with 40 normal persons, matched for age, education, and intelligence. The subjects were asked to select the best of four correct definitions on a vocabulary test, with each definition representing either class, example, description, or function. The schizophrenic selected more function and example definitions, whereas the normal subjects preferred class definitions.

One can speculate that careful, experimental study of verbal behavior may provide the basis for a much deeper understanding of personality and adjustment than now exists. But comprehensive analyses of verbal behavior, such as that occurring in an interview, are laborious and expensive. It is likely that studies of verbal behavior will continue to require a high degree of effort, but the significance and value of the findings will increase with refined techniques.

Physiological and Organic Measures

Personality characteristics and emotional maladjustment are frequently associated with physiological dysfunction, organic damage, or bodily structural atypicalities. The tense, overactive victim of hyperthyroid ism, the epileptic whose seizures are the product of brain scar tissue, and the saddle-nosed mongoloid child are obvious cases in point. Such physical indicators are often direct reflections of the personality variables under study and, at times, are causally related to them. Thus they are, potentially, more objective, pertinent, and sensitive, and simpler than the measures in common use. Indeed, there is ample evidence that the relationship of personality to such indicators is often quite close. But there are problems. For example, if the symptoms are treated without the investigator's knowledge, the symptoms may disappear, leaving unchanged the conflict or whatever personality facet is under study. Thus, one may try to find identifying characteristics of anxiety neurosis by measuring eye blink rate, tics, tremors, etc., in a group of anxiety neurotics and in a control group. If, however, the anxiety-ridden patients have been given tranquilizers, they may blink, tic, and tremble no differently from the controls. Today, especially, it is almost impossible to find schizophrenic patients who are untranquilized and unshocked. Another problem is that the symptoms should relate directly and meaningfully to the personality characteristic under scrutiny. Tremors, for example, are often associated with anxiety reactions; yet various subjective and objective measures will sometimes indicate that the anxiety-neurotic patient is much improved, although the tremor remains. Whether the consequence of functional autonomy, a chance relationship, or sheer obstinacy on the part of the patient, the tremor persists, to the confusion of the earnest researcher who was using it as a response measure.

Symptom removal, of course, may be of prime importance to the patient. He comes for help because of general tension and skipped heartbeats, for example, and departs reasonably satisfied when his tension is relieved and the extra systoles have disappeared. It matters little to the patient, nor, in most cases, to the practitioner, whether pill, palaver, or neither produced the change. But it matters a great deal to the experimentalist, for he must know why, the answer to which is the reason for his professional existence. Curiously, while the practical treatment situation may offer pitfalls for the unwary researcher, the researcher himself often has his own blind spots. Do measurements taken in a laboratory setting, for example, apply to clinical problems? Then, when an actual treatment setting is employed, can the measures taken be generalized to other situations at work, play, or home? They may indeed, but few investigators have made any attempt to check this.

Still another question concerns the extent to which physiological measures may be meaningfully related to personality characteristics. Wenger in a careful study of a wide range of physiological variables with a large number of subjects, found difficulty in locating any significant correlations among the measures he used. In Part III of the present volume, Psychophysiology, the chapters by Brady, Dews, Malmo and Pribram describe a great many studies dealing with physiological and organic measures which relate to personality. Thus, the following studies are presented chiefly as examples of the kind of measures which have been used for assessment purposes, not as an exhaustive review.

Most research dealing with physiological and organic factors in relation to personality has been concerned with deviant personality states and personality change rather than with the dimensions of the normal personality. Thus a great deal has been published on skin conductance, brain waves, muscle tension, etc., in schizophrenia, but very little on such measures as applied to general sociability or similar traits, as they occur in normal people. The measures actually used vary from direct, simple observation to elaborate records obtained from complex and elegant apparatus. In an observational study, for example, Altus found that enuresis and constipation were indicators of personality disturbance among illiterate soldiers. Some additional examples of such simple measures are worthy of consideration. Goddard and Doll used hand preference in studies of mental retardation, and found a limited relationship between left-hand preference and feeblemindedness. Olson measured nervous habits in children by recording the number of times the children picked their noses or put fingers into their mouths during a series of five-minute observation periods. More recently, Meyer, Bahrick and Fitts tried to measure anxiety by determining eye blink frequency during short time periods, on the hypothesis that blink rate was positively related to anxiety. Although more complex in the sense of chemistry laboratory technique, direct observation was also employed in Fischer's report that a component in the urine of acute schizophrenics was of much greater toxicity than that of normal control subjects.

Examples of measures obtained through the use of apparatus are many and varied. One of the instruments in longest use is the psychogalvanometer, which has been used to measure galvanometric skin responses (GSR) in a variety of settings. Studies employing the GSR as measures of personality facets have frequently had disappointing results; yet there continues to be something tantalizing about them. Herr and Kobler, for example, tried to distinguish between normal and neurotic subjects by means of the GSR with little success. Nevertheless, the greater variability of the neurotics and the direction of mean response change for certain empirically identified stimulus words indicated to the authors that it should eventually be possible to differentiate the two groups. The GSR varies with the therapist's permissiveness in a treatment situation, according to Dittes, and thus seems to Dittes to represent a measure of anxiety or "mobilization" against any sign of punishment by the therapist.

The GSR magnitude of deflection does seem to bear a close relationship to subjects' estimates of the intensity of their experience and should eventually prove to be a valuable research tool. McCurdy makes this point in a highly readable review of GSR literature which should be a "must" for any researcher interested in this field. He recomputed data from a wide variety of studies and found the correlations of the intensity of experience and GSR magnitude of deflection to range from .45 to 1.00, with an average of .75, certainly an impressive relationship. The problem for personality assessment seems to be one of using the GSR appropriately. As Eysenck observed, little progress is likely to be made until fundamental problems of measurement are resolved.

Like the GSR studies, research with the electroencephalograph (EEG), electrocardiograph (EKG), and instruments designed to measure other physical responses such as muscle tension, skin temperature, and capillary blood saturation have provided provocative if inconclusive data. Faure, for example, found in a study of anxiety patients that the degree of anxiety roughly paralleled the degree of perturbance of cerebral electrical potentials when a light was applied. In the more severe cases of anxiety the EEG was not modified by opening or closing the eyes. Morselli investigated a case of multiple personality with the EEG. During abnormal periods, the EEG records resembled those of Pentothal prenarcosis-that is, increased amplitude and irregular rhythm characteristics of partial sleep. When the normal personality was dominant, the EEG record was also normal. A hundred psychotic patients with various diagnoses were examined with the EEG by Lyketsos, Belinson, and Gibbs. They found no slow wave foci, and the EEG sleep patterns of the psychotics were lower in voltage than those for normal controls. Levy and Dennard also used a hundred subjects in a study of the EEG records of penitentiary inmates compared to those obtained for a normal population. They found a significantly larger proportion of abnormal records among the prisoners, and some evidence which suggested that relatively good personality structure was related to normal EEG's.

Other measures, such as recordings of muscular tension, have been used in relation to personality adjustment. When hostility themes are discussed, for example, a high level of muscular tension is recorded in the forearms but discussion of sexual conflict is associated with similar tension in the legs. In another study of muscle tension, Stennett found that when motivating conditions are varied from low to high levels, muscle tension and palmar sweating also vary systematically with the changes in motivating conditions.

Some studies have employed highly specific bodily areas for measurement purposes. Mowrer, Light, Luria and Seleny, for example, measured fingertip sweating and found a relationship of this response to patient's self-ratings of tension during psychotherapy. Anxiety as identified by psychological tests, however, does not seem to relate to palmar sweating according to studies by Lotsof and Downing and by Calvin, McGuigan, Tyrrell, and Soyars. Fingertip temperature as measured by a thermocouple was used by Flecker to demonstrate that a rise in finger temperature was associated with emotional security and a drop with states of conflict. The heartbeat has also been used as a measure in therapy situations. Di Mascio, Boyd, Greenblatt, and Solomon found a correlation of +.79 between patients' and therapists' heart rate during the initial stages of the interview but -.44 for the final stages. They also reported the rather provocative findings that one psychotherapist always produced a lower heart rate in all three subjects of one of their experiments.

Many studies of physiological and organic response measures in relation to personality could be reviewed. But the foregoing sampling gives at least the flavor of the kind of investigations reported within this area. Eventually-but a long time ahead-personality may be expressed in terms of blood and tissue components, the structure of organs, and the functioning of body cells. Somehow the present efforts seem vaguely reminiscent of the medieval alchemist's search for the philosopher's stone. Many investigators seem implicitly, if unconsciously searching for the one measure which will be the foot rule for the personality trait under study. This is in no way intended to belittle their efforts; for some research has indeed come encouragingly within view of such a foot rule. What is needed in the near future is an inspired theoretician who can assimilate the varied research findings and come out with a clear-cut general principle. Then a basic science of personality will emerge; it will probably introduce measurements based on chemistry and physics, not psychology.

Environmental and Achievement Measures

How one behaves in the social milieu is probably the major criterion used by others in appraising personality. The alcoholic, the schizophrenic, the juvenile delinquent, are commonly first identified by their social behavior. The same is true of positively valued responses such as the man who keeps his head in an emergency or who is liked by others and elected to high office. Praise, punishment, or treatment is meted out chiefly on the basis of behavior in the social environment. But if behavior in this context is the criterion employed for personality assessment by the general public, it is not often the criterion used in research studies when measuring therapeutic gain or personality change. Effective psychotherapy, of course, should produce altered responses in the problem area; that is, if treatment is to have real meaning, the chronic alcoholic should have quit drinking, the juvenile delinquent should have ceased his offenses, the oft-discharged worker ought to keep a job. Take the schizophrenic who no longer thinks he is God; there has been a remission of symptom, true, but then he may be sent home to mope in idleness. For the clinical record he is listed as successfully treated; in actuality the treatment is successful only in the sense of "off our backs and on the family's." The truer test is whether he can return to work and acceptably perform his duties. This observation minimizes neither the value of partial success in therapeutic effort nor the importance of even slight improvement. But the main goal of therapy is to return the patient to society as a useful, contributing, and self-sustaining member, although this admittedly is not possible for most patients at present.

A wide variety of environmental and achievement measures have been used at times to assess personality change, but their use has not been common. The problem is that such measures are both expensive and difficult to obtain. Job promotions, salary increases, absenteeism, accident rates, participation in social activities, to name but a few, are indeed useful criteria when properly employed. But to gather such data accurately over a period of years is exceedingly difficult. Former patients move to other cities, change jobs, exaggerate some information items and conceal others because of shame. Yet, if full information cannot be obtained over a period of time, some data on environmental and achievement correlates of personality can usually be assembled for assessment purposes.

Thus Friedman evaluated the effects of short-term therapy with 50 patients who complained of a phobia for travel by ascertaining whether, after treatment, they were actually able to travel. Twelve were unchanged, 15 showed improvement, and 23 were able to travel freely. One might, of course, like answers to other questions, such as whether other symptoms later replaced the phobia for travel. But the report at least measures improvement on one environmental criterion, and this is clearly a step in the right direction.

Environmental and achievement correlates to personality are not yet widely used, and the application of such criterion measures can be critized when they are used. Yet, such approaches are likely to provide the most useful criteria for many research situations. It seems appropriate, therefore, to review some of the investigations in this area.

Teuber and Powers wondered how effective psychotherapy would be with potential delinquents. With this question in mind, they matched a non treatment control group with similar youngsters who were given psychotherapy. The number of court appearances over a period of time was totaled and compared for the two groups of potential delinquents. There were no significant differences.

Fox evaluated a prison counseling program by a variety of ratings and measures such as work records, school stability, financial budgeting, and reports from chaplains, cell block officers, and work supervisors, as well as successful discharge from, or violation of, parole. The counseled group did significantly better than the control group in terms of these environmental criteria. A similarly realistic study is that by Ludwig and Ranson who evaluated the success of treatment for combat-induced NP disability by the percentage of servicemen who could return to full combat duty. This is an obviously important criterion, because return to active duty as a kitchen hand, for example, is quite different from return to full combat duty.

Behavior in an institutional setting may be meaningful for evaluating the progress of a treatment program. Thus Cowden, Zax, Hague, and Finney evaluated the improvement made in a group of patients receiving group psychotherapy and chlorpromazine as compared to a non treatment control group. As criteria for improvement, they used frequency counts of the times a patient required neural wet packs or electroconvulsive shock, engaged in fights or was transferred to less disturbed wards. Those receiving group therapy and chlorpromazine showed more improvement than the controls. Raush, Dittman and Taylor, using similar environmental events assessed change resulting from treatment administered to children in a residential setting. They standardized observations on the children's behavior during meal times, play periods, and arts-and-crafts sessions. With such measures they found that the most significant changes occurred in the children's relationship to adults, while their relationships with peers changed relatively little. These studies confirm the assumption that how an individual behaves as he moves about in his particular environment is a significant factor in the appraisal of adjustment.

In a study covering a seventeen-year period, Thorne found that the important measures of psychological health included a stable work history, broad range of vocational and avocational interests, socially approved habits such as sobriety and thrift, and, of course, freedom from chronic mental disorders. Interestingly and perhaps deterministically, the social classes which are less likely to meet Thorne's criteria are the ones which have the highest incidence of mental disorders. As Hollingshead and Redlich noted, not only do the members of the lower social strata contribute more NP patients but the treatment they get is likely to be different from that received by other classes. The lower classes are much more likely to receive electroconvulsive shock; the middle and upper classes more frequently receive psychotherapy. Kahn, Pollack and Fink reported similar findings in an investigation of type of treatment of mental patients as related to age, education, and birthplace. The older, less educated, and foreign-born were more likely to receive electroconvulsive shock than other patients. Like Hollingshead and Redlich, they found that the patients who resembled therapists in their higher social background were more frequently given psychotherapy.

There is a problem in how to handle these measures and in understanding what they mean. As Berg observed, "The use of environmental or achievement correlates requires a value judgment on the part of the investigator, namely, that the observed change validly indicates a better or poorer adjustment. At times this may be misleading. Lower academic grades, for example, may not signify poorer adjustment but merely that 'boy has met girl,' often a healthier symptom than higher grades." The same might be said of the ulcer ridden, tremor-wracked sales executive who takes a lower paying job but thereby achieves better personal adjustment. In our culture we regard higher grades and increased salaries as signs of progress, but they do not always indicate better emotional equilibrium.

Problems exist not only in interpretation, but also in obtaining certain kinds of information. Information may be unavailable either because of policy or because it is unknown. Thus, company regulations may forbid supplying information on disciplinary action, absenteeism, or reprimands about an employee who was formerly under treatment. In a small business, after a year or two, personnel changes and an absence of formal records may similarly prevent the gathering of accurate data. Worse, an informant may deliberately mislead an investigator by indicating that an employee left voluntarily, perhaps for a better job, when actually he was told to find another job. But the informant is unwilling to prejudice what he regards as a new start for the former employee. Then, too, there are the limitations that the investigator must impose upon himself. In our culture many persons cling to medieval ideas about mental illness. Thus the investigator may have to exercise so much discretion in approaching those in contact with a discharged patient that it is hardly worth the effort, particularly in view of the difficulties even the most cautious inquiry may create for the ex-patient.

In general, the first caution in the use of environmental and achievement correlates would be that those selected are valid indications of improved adjustment. Second, multiple criteria are likely to be much more meaningful than single measures. Finally, the information sources must be closely scrutinized for maximum accuracy of report and for complete protection of the former patient. With these conditions met, it is probable that the most meaningful measures of therapeutic gain will be obtained if the measures can be repeated over a fairly lengthy period under conditions of before, during, and after treatment.

Experimentally Induced Personality Change

The experimentally induced personality change requires that the changes or abnormal states be deliberately created, preferably along a single dimension. Various techniques have been used to produce appropriate changes for experimental study: role playing, in which an abnormal state such as mental retardation is simulated by a normal person; psychological stress, intended to arouse fear, anger, frustration, loss of self-esteem, etc.; noxious stimuli, either actual or impending, employed in the form of electric shock, etc., used to produce conflict or chaotic states in the subject; deprivation or alteration of stimuli, in which an absence or modification of stimuli causes behavioral changes; drugs and biochemical components, in which pharmaceutical and biochemical preparations create anxiety, depression, symptoms of mental disorder, etc.; reactivation of a dormant conflict or state of maladjustment, whereby a once-troublesome adjustment problem is again made a source of conflict.

In all of these procedures, measures are (or should be) taken before, during, and after the experimental condition, and any or all of the previously described methods of assessment may be used for this purpose-that is, rating, and psychological tests. Strictly speaking, such induction of personality change is a research design rather than a particular assessment method. Nevertheless, as an approach to the experimental study of personality it has great potential for definitive research. We might prophesy that the major breakthroughs in personality research will be brought about by these approaches in which personality changes are experimentally induced. But these procedures must be accompanied by caution and elaborate safeguards in order to avoid public misunderstanding of these techniques.

Much of the earlier work in this area was done with animals. Maier described a series of experiments in which he produced abnormal behavior in the rat by such techniques as forcing the animals to either brave a blast of air or jump across an open space and fall into a net. Landis and Hunt also summarized a long series of studies in which they used human as well as animal subjects in their investigation of the startle pattern. By means of sudden, intense stimulation, they produced catastrophic behavior in the organisms and measured the ensuing flexion (startle) response. While they produced a temporary upheaval which may legitimately be termed a state of maladjustment, their interest was limited to the startle pattern manifestations and did not include other possible associated personality effects.

Role Playing or Simulation

In role playing, the subject is instructed to respond to some measuring instrument, such as a psychological test, as if he had a particular personality characteristic or type of maladjustment. An essential condition, of course, is that the subjects have the necessary information to do a good job in their role. Usually, the experimenter has some purpose in mind other than the apparent or announced one. Thus Gough had persons familiar with clinical diagnosis simulate severe psychoneurosis and then paranoid schizophrenia when responding to the MMPI. He found that his subjects under such instructions produced MMPI profiles quite similar to those of genuine patients. Although interested in this finding, Gough was more interested in whether such faking could be detected. He found that the MMPI F, or validity, score minus the K, or test-taking attitude, score provided a means of detecting the fakers.

Using a similar approach, Goldstein and Pollaczek instructed subjects of normal intelligence to respond to intelligence test items as if they were mentally retarded. The responses thus obtained in both studies were then compared with the test responses of bona fide mental defectives. The malingerers showed definite patterns in their faking; for, while they were able to obtain low intelligence scores, how they answered various items provided a sound basis for detection. They missed many easy items which the true feebleminded cases were able to answer correctly; at times, they missed other items in a systematic manner-that is, as if they figured out the right answer and then deviated from it in a standard fashion. Both Goldstein and Pollaczek were each able then to prepare "malingering" keys for detecting faking on intelligence tests.

In another facet of role playing, the subject is not instructed in his role but rather assumes it voluntarily, usually for purposes of gaining some personal advantage. A clerical employee studied by Paterson, for example, strongly desired a promotion to a personnel position, for which he was given both the Kuder and the Strong interest inventories. Although the employee slanted his responses to favor the promotion he wished to attain, the test data nevertheless indicated that the employee's interests were basically in clerical, not in personnel activities. Paterson's interest lay in observing whether the Kuder or the Strong was more easily faked in such situations; of the two, the Kuder appeared to be the more easily slanted. However, although situations in which the self-interest of subjects lead them to malinger are not common, it seems like that such self-imposed roles with natural conditions of motivation behind them could provide the framework for useful studies of personality change.

Psychological Stress

In experimental stress situations, the subject is placed under pressure, and measures taken before and after the stress condition. Sarason found that subjects identified operationally as high in manifest anxiety performed poorly on a serial learning task when faced with pronounced threat of failure, whereas low anxiety subjects were not adversely affected. The high and low anxiety groups showed no differences when threat of failure was not present. Heath examined the effects of anxiety upon the intellectual performance of schizophrenic subjects by using test content constructed around anxiety themes. He found that there were individual thresholds for the appearance of anxiety responses in such subjects, and that severe anxiety had a disorganizing effect for the performance of intellectual tasks. Grinker, Sabshin, Hamburg, Board, Basowitz, Korchin, Persky, and Chevalier also employed psychiatric patients under conditions of stress in the form of interviews which, in non reassuring fashion, probed the patients' most sensitive areas of conflict. The investigators were unable to control the degree of anxiety thus aroused nor were they able to grade the stimuli in relation to the anxiety produced. The possible forms of stress which have been employed at one time or another are many and varied, ranging from a physical examination to requiring subjects to cut off the head of a live rat. Whatever type of stress is used, it is essential that the stimuli utilized actually represent stress for the subject. A number of situations which would be regarded as distasteful, embarrassing, or threatening for the experimenter are nothing of the sort for many subjects.

Noxious Stimuli

To the extent that potentially harmful stimuli are impending but not applied, the technique of noxious stimuli is essentially the same as the stress procedures already described. Perhaps it matters little whether the noxious stimuli are actually applied or merely threatened, since the effect upon the subject may be much the same in either case.

Threat alone should not be underestimated; young men in good health, as in the military services, have been known to faint at the prospect of a hypodermic injection. Schachter, for example, subjected hypertensive and normotensive patients to various situations designed to arouse fear, anger, and pain. He found that a significantly greater rise in blood pressure occurred in the hypertensive patients as compared to the controls. Furthermore, the hypertensive subjects gave more overt indications of fear and anger than the normotensives. At times, conflicting results are reported for similar situations. For example, whereas Sarason found that subjects high in manifest anxiety performed relatively poorly in a serial learning task when threatened with failure, Silverman and Blitz found, by contrast, that high anxiety subjects who were threatened with shock did not exhibit poorer learning performance in learning tasks. Perhaps such differences occur as a function of the seriousness with which the subjects take the purported threatening condition. In any event, it would be desirable to have data on the nature and conditions of noxious stimuli. The recent burgeoning of space medicine research may well provide some of the needed information. Human subjects have been stressed with gravitational pull, high and low temperatures, confinement to small spaces, loud noises, etc. However, although such data are likely to be useful, personality measures are not usually included when appraising these stress effects.

Deprivation or Alteration of Stimuli

In deprivation or alteration of stimulus studies, the subject is deprived of sensory stimulation by some means, or the normal stimulus conditions are altered in some manner. Bexton, Heron, and Scott, among others, used a soundproof room for this purpose, Lily immersed snorkel-equipped subjects in a tank of water. All sensory input was not eliminated, of course, since certain tactile and kinesthetic sensations could not be completely cut off; yet the results were striking. The subjects experienced auditory and visual hallucinations, and were unable to follow a connected line of thought. At times, a blank period occurred in which all mental content appeared to be absent. Certain of these effects appeared to linger in attenuated form for as long as twenty-four hours after the experiment ended. Stimulus alteration has also been achieved in other ways, such as in the use of tilting-chair and artificial horizon studies with airplane pilots or in the auditory feedback research on speech. Indeed, almost any form of illusion or change in stimulus property could be employed to study various facets of personality, although such has not often been the case. The usual measure taken is a decrement in performance, as on a verbal learning task, a pursuit rotor, or other perceptual motor activity. But the applications to personality study are both obvious and promising.

Several interesting studies have been reported wherein the usual conditions of auditory stimulation were modified, although the particular stimulus properties remained unchanged. Hassel, Magaret and Cameron had a group of college students compose a five minute story based upon one of the pictures in the Thematic Apperception Test (TAT). For half the group the stories were tape-recorded and then, while the subjects sought to composed a second TAT story, the first story which each had composed was played back to them by means of earphones. The other half of the group composed two stories, one after the other, without interference. It was found that the distraction resulted in a significantly greater amount of scattered speech by the subjects, but with increased meaningfulness in the story itself. Fairbanks and Guttman have used a somewhat analogous but more powerful technique in their studies of language disorganization. Their approach required the subjects to speak into a recorder; then, after a delay of 0, .1, .2, .4, and .8 seconds, the subjects heard what they had just uttered repeated through earphones while they read aloud a prose passage. The delay produced marked articulatory disturbances, phonetically illogical substitutions, and additions which were repetitive and apparently unpurposeful.

Drugs and Biochemical Components

Pharmaceutical preparations such as drugs or biochemical are also used to change adjustment or personality characteristics. The assumptions underlying research of this sort are soundly based, for ordinary experience with the effects of such drugs as alcohol, barbiturates, or Benzedrine offer ample evidence of their capacity for modifying behavior. Anxiety states, depressions, hallucinations, have all been produced by the use of the appropriate drug. Because of the intense public interest in chemotherapy as a possible "cure" for mental disorder, the professional literature available in this field during the past decade is enormous, although many of the studies are poorly controlled and must be regarded as inconclusive. In general, what have been called miracle drugs in the public press are far less miraculous in their effects than the initial enthusiasm for them would have indicated. They are useful, yes, but neither the key nor necessarily the ultimate answer to personality aberration.

At the level of clinical description, however, a number of personality disorders are indistinguishable from symptomatology produced by drugs or toxic conditions. As Hoskins observed, schizoid reactions can be produced by bulbocapnine, mescaline, alcohol, morphine, and even by breathing air of reduced oxygen content. Experimentally, the most widely used drug for producing psychopathological states is probably lysergic acid diethylamide (LSD). According to Salvatore and Hyde, this drug produces a series of behavioral changes which begin with bodily symptoms and anxiety reactions followed by perceptual distortions and feelings of unreality. The final stage appears to be characterized by attempts to cope with the feeling of unreality, during which various degrees of mental confusion result. After approximately six hours the symptoms dissipate. In a critical review of LSD research, Clark questions whether the LSD-induced experience is the same in form as any known natural psychotic state. He notes that most studies either omit or have inadequate control groups, that observations are often unsystematic, and that the experimenter and the subject may at times be biased, because both have knowledge of the drug's behavioral effects.

The criticisms Clark leveled at LSD studies may with equal justice be applied to research on glutamic acid. On the basis of reports which indicated that learning performance in rats could be improved by the administration of glutamic acid, this drug was used in attempts to raise the level of intellectual functioning in human subjects. The reports were conflicting; however in an analysis of the various studies, Astin and Ross showed that positive findings with respects to raised intelligence after glutamic acid administration were definitely associated with a lack of control data.

Another technique employs blood components of the victims of psychopathological conditions. Heath and his colleagues have used taraxein, a protein substance which is obtained from the blood of schizophrenic patients to produce schizophrenia experimentally.

These investigators injected taraxein in nonpsychotic prison inmates who volunteered for the study. All twenty subjects developed primary symptoms of schizophrenia, including autism, thought blocking, and depersonalization, as well as secondary symptoms such as delusions and auditory hallucinations. They also employed a rapid transfusion of blood from schizophrenic to normal subjects and reported that the transfused subjects exhibited mild schizophrenic symptoms which lasted for an hour or less. Freedman and Ginsberg reversed this procedure and replaced about 60 per cent of the blood of schizophrenic patients with blood from normal donors. Three adult schizophrenics showed no change and a slight improvement was noted in one schizophrenic child. Hoagland attempted to duplicate the Heath researches with taraxein, but he was unsuccessful. Generally, the results of studies in this area have been conflicting and thus far inconclusive. It seems likely that the research design is faulty in many of these investigations and that inadequate, qualitative assessment is employed in place of more quantitative measurement of behavioral change. There may very well be something of critical, perhaps of ultimate significance for the understanding of personality and maladjustment in future research which employs drugs or biochemical components. Certainly hormonal and other changes do seem to be present in psychopathological states. However, whether this is due to the disorder, a function of long hospitalization, or something else is not clear. Controls are needed but they are often difficult to attain. Just as an aside, it may be noted that it is frequently very difficult to locate patients who have not been given drugs or perhaps electroconvulsive shock treatment prior to NP hospital admission, so common has such prehospitalization practice become-all of which points up the pressing need for controls.

Reactivation of a Dormant Conflict or State of Maladjustment

The reactivation of a previous conflict presumably permits study and/or treatment with the aim of understanding the processes involved and, perhaps, testing the efficacy of a treatment method. The technique is rarely used, probably because of the obvious difficulties and possible dangers involved. Indeed, the only carefully designed study is probably that by Keet, which dealt with such minuscule problem areas that the technique may have limited applications at best. Keet used word association tests to identify conflict areas and then treated the miniature conflict by nondirective and directive procedures. The directive or interpretive techniques were found to be far more effective than nondirective methods-so much better that several investigators were led to replicate his study. However, replication was never accomplished. Merrill, for example, did not find any difference between the two methods of treatment which would confirm Keet 's results. Apart from the lack of support for Keet 's results, the research design he used is ingenious and worth studying.

Theoretical Explanations of Assessment

The material reviewed thus far demonstrates that a wide range of stimulus materials can be employed to produce a broad variety of responses which, in turn, can be used to assess personality and personality change. Furthermore, the evidence cited is but a small sampling of many thousands of similar studies. True, some of the assessment techniques described are considerably more effective than others for purposes of clinical prediction; but virtually all of them predict or otherwise identify personality characteristics at least to some degree. Hundreds of response measures have been used in thousands of personality investigations. Some of the measures do an adequate and needed clinical job of assessment, whereas the others predict only somewhat better than chance. Now, with so many and such varied techniques having at least some value for personality appraisal, the question remains: "Why? Why do so many different methods predict behavior?" In addition to the familiar inkblots, pictures, or verbal test items, one can employ the Archimedes spiral aftereffect, the autokinetic phenomenon, hand preference, musical sounds, meaningless sounds, amount of body sway and myriad other measures; yet all of them have varying degrees of value. In a discussion called "The Unimportance of Test Item Content", it has been asserted that virtually any stimulus material and any sense modality could be employed for purposes of personality measurement. Not all such materials are of equal value-as, for example, not every item of the MMPI is just as good as any other for measuring the Hy (hysteria) or some other scale. But one could find a sound or an abstract design or some other stimulus material which would predict as well as a particular MMPI item for a given scale. In that sense, then, a particular type of test item content is unimportant.

In attempting to explain why personality assessment devices do measure, the oldest explanation is, by implication, that of face validity. Test materials were chosen because they obviously related to the variable under study; hence if one were interested in emotionality, he prepared items which inquired whether the subject was prone to "lose his temper easily" or whether he was "calm in emergencies," etc. Thus, although test item face validity was not systematized as an explanation of why psychological tests measured personality, the content used and the procedures followed in developing the older personality tests demonstrated that face validity was the basis for such assessment. During the last twenty-five years, although preoccupation with face validity was still evident in item construction, the actual basis for determining the value of a particular item gradually became empirical in orientation. Accordingly, a test item dealing with reading habits might be retained in a neurotic scale, even though its content seemed to be unrelated to neuroticism, because it was a differentiating factor. Another item with obvious face validity, such as a question about how often one felt jittery, would be rejected if it failed to differentiate neurotic from normal subjects to some degree. The usefulness of an item, therefore, was decided empirically, a simple modus operandi, yet one which was not always fully understood. Hutt, for example, asserted that structured personality tests were based on the assumption that the items would have the same meaning for all subjects who took the test, a misunderstanding for which Meehl took Hutt sharply to task.

Under the onslaught of empirical approaches, interest in face validity was no longer paramount as the basis for constructing personality tests, leaving the question still open as to why personality tests measure. During the past decade, three explanations have been proposed as a first and partial step in resolving this question. These are explanations based upon (1) Content and Style, (2) the Social Desirability Variable and (3) the Deviation Hypothesis.

Content and style in personality assessment: In studying behavior, one may examine the content (what is said or done) and the style or mode (how it is said or done). In denying a request, for example, a person may say "no" in soft, level tones unaccompanied by other bodily activity, or he may roar "no" while glaring balefully and leaning tensely forward. Jackson and Messick have remarked that although these two response characteristics are conceptually distinct, style is often overlooked. Therefore these writers propose that measures of response style, rather than content, are more likely to provide for adequate assessment of personality, and that such measurements may bridge the gap between personality theory and personality measurement. Most of the evidence they offer is based upon various studies of the California S scale which purports to measure authoritarianism, but actually seems to measure acquiescence. Jackson and Messick and Jackson, Messick and Solley, among other students of the problem, have shown that style rather than content is of chief importance in the F scale. These writers have been interested primarily in acquiescence as a characteristic response style; however, by extension they could apply their concept to other personality assessment techniques and thus offer an explanation of why and how various techniques measure. Cronbach has discussed various response style characteristics (he called them response sets) as they occur in psychological tests. In addition to acquiescence, Cronbach described a number of other styles-for example, tendency to gamble, evasiveness-however, he urged that such "sets" be identified and then eliminated in tests because of their influence on reliability and validity. Jackson and Messick propose to use, rather than eliminate, such response styles. Thus far, not too much evidence about the value of response styles has been accumulated, but it seems reasonable to predict that Jackson and Messick's confidence in such response characteristics will be justified. Certainly a large number of behavioral facets can be examined and tested experimentally within the content versus style framework.

The social desirability variable: Edwards has contended that almost any statement or item concerned with personality can be characterized in terms of its position on a single dimension. He calls this dimension the social desirability undesirability variable, and further states that it appears to be the most important single dimension on which to locate personality statements. In his book on the social desirability variable in relation to personality assessment, he presents a great deal of evidence on psychological tests to support his contention. For example, Klett found a relationship of .88 between social desirability scale values obtained for psychotic patients and college students, indicating that these subjects were rating the items in much the same way. Similarly, Hanley obtained correlations of .82 and .89, respectively, between probability of endorsement and social desirability ratings for samples of items from the MMPI D (symptomatic depression) and Sc (schizophrenia) scales.

With such evidence in mind, Edwards constructed a Personal Preference Schedule in which, he believes, the social desirability variable has been controlled. The studies of Silver and Kelleher support this belief. However, Goodstein and Heilbrun and Wiggins and Rumrill have raised doubts concerning the significance and pureness of this variable. Whatever the outcome of future studies on the SD variable, it seems likely that the approach is too narrow to explain more than a limited number of assessment methods. As noted earlier, an investigator may employ spiral after effects, autokinetic phenomena, eye blink rate, and other stimulus response conditions for assessing personality-all of them techniques whose effectiveness would not seem to be explained by the social desirability variable.

The deviation hypothesis: An approach which attempts to embrace a much broader spectrum of behavior is the deviation hypothesis. This conception is not limited to an explanation of why various techniques are able to measure, in varying degree, familiar dimensions of personality such as sociability, or psychopathological conditions such as schizophrenia. Although such personality facets are included in the formulation of the deviation hypothesis, many other behavior patterns, such as academic over- and underachievement, accident proneness, mental retardation, immaturity, and senescence are also included. Of the immense repertoire of all possible responses, according to this view, many responses are regarded as clustering or hanging together to form various patterns. Certain of these patterns are different or deviant in the sense that they are uncommon and may be objectively identified by simple statistical methods. They are not necessarily deviant in the sense of psychopathology; rather, they are deviant in the sense of a departure from the modal pattern, just as the literal meaning of abnormal is away from the norm or common pattern. Hence, a surgeon, an 80-year-old man, and a schizophrenic would each be deviant because most people are not surgeons, 80 years old, nor schizophrenics. What is important is that such deviant patterns be significant in some manner and be identified in an objective, operationally clean fashion. The deviation hypothesis makes the assumption that deviant responses are general; and if a deviant behavior pattern can be validly identified in a critical area of behavior (i.e., psychotic reactions), deviant behavior patterns can be identified in non critical areas (i.e., responses to test items). This hypothesis has been stated as follows: "Deviant response patterns tend to be general; hence, those deviant behavior patterns which are significant for abnormality (atypicalness) and thus regarded as symptoms (ear marks or signs), are associated with other deviant response patterns which are in non critical areas of behavior and which are not regarded as symptoms of personality aberration (nor as indicators, signs, ear marks)." This does not mean, of course, that every response made by a deviant person will be deviant; obviously we are all deviant in a few areas. Yet most of our responses are quite like those of other people. But certain small patterns of deviant responses in a significant area of behavior (for example, schizophrenia) do appear to be associated with response patterns in unimportant areas of behavior (for example, marking a particular MMPI item true as opposed to false). If deviant responses are general in the sense outlined above the deviation hypothesis would explain why such a vast array of materials can be used to assess personality and other aspects of behavior.

3

Operant Techniques

Introduction

Traditionally areas of human pathology received clinical attention long before the laboratory could make its contribution. Human misery makes its demands immediately felt, and science is slow. This is as true of behavioral pathology as it has been of liver disease or endocrine malfunction or any of the other more obviously biological problems to which man is subject. The clinical psychologist is impatient; the press of immediacy impels him to build his clinical house as best he can before an experimental foundation is available.

From simple analogy with the various medical disciplines we can expect that an appropriate laboratory science will indeed prove useful to the behavioral clinician. No more subtle argument than this need be made for the desirability of an experimental foundation. Similarly, we can expect the clinician to welcome this help when it does arrive. But what kinds of help is he to expect from the laboratory?

There are a number of areas of potential contact between the clinic and the laboratory: investigative techniques, basic research and theory, classification and diagnosis, and therapeutic practices. I shall discuss each of these areas and, wherever possible, shall provide detailed examples selected from the available literature.

Investigative Techniques

One of the claims of experimental psychology is that it can help sharpen the methodological and evaluative tools of clinical investigation. Experimentalists have offered the clinician two major contributions: the control group, and statistics. As a result, analysis of variance is now almost as common a tool in clinical behavioral research as is the stethoscope in clinical cardiac research.

I have argued elsewhere, and at some length, that control groups and statistical evaluation of data are among the least desirable features of much current laboratory research. The same may be said of clinical research except, of course, where the interest is in normative or epidemiological problems. Clinically derived knowledge is, in the last analysis, subject to the same pragmatic criteria that are used to evaluate laboratory findings. When enough practitioners of research, diagnosis, or therapy have been able to replicate or use a finding, that finding then becomes an established datum, a bit of knowledge.

It is in using the results of his research that the clinician will recognize the sterility of statistical evaluation. For he cannot, in his practice, deal with a mythical average individual, a group composite. He cannot diagnose a group nor can he treat one-a statistical group, that is to say. He must apply his research findings to individuals.

What else does experimental psychology have to offer the clinician? My brief criticism of the relevance of statistical methodology leads directly to a discussion of operant conditioning techniques, with which I shall be concerned in the remainder of this chapter. The methodology of operant conditioning has several features that the clinical investigator will find congenial: It obtains its data from the individual; it uses the individual as his own control; it evaluates data in terms of its replicability and utility; it uses techniques that have species generality; it examines instances of variability. But most relevant of all are the contributions made by operant conditioning to our fund of techniques of behavioral manipulation. Such techniques are the unique province of a science of behavior, and if experimental psychology cannot provide these the clinician may justifiably conclude that his experimental foundations have yet to be built.

The bulk of operant conditioning work has been carried out with species lower than man on the phylogenetic scale. This has undoubtedly contributed to the existing gap between clinician and experimentalist. Furthermore, the basic experimental interest has been in normal, rather than pathological, behavioral processes. The assumptions have been that (1) the increased rigor of experimental control permitted by work with lower animals makes it possible to discover and isolate behavioral processes whose relevance to humans may then be assessed under more complex circumstances; and (2) an understanding of normal behavior is a prerequisite for the adequate evaluation of malfunctioning behavioral processes. How well have these assumptions stood up?

I shall begin by summarizing the technical foundation that has been built upon animal studies, and illustrate the techniques by describing some of the extensions that have been made to normal human behavior in the laboratory. The exposition is intended to serve three functions: The first is to indicate to the clinical investigator some of the techniques that are available to him for manipulating a subject's behavior in controlled investigation. These are basic tools with which every student of behavior should be acquainted, for they give him direct access to his subject matter. The second function is to indicate the range in which the techniques have been found applicable to human subjects. Not all of them have been so applied, and certain difficulties have been encountered, but there is a sufficient weight of evidence to demonstrate that the animal work is both practical and relevant in principle to human behavior; I shall emphasize the technical practicality in this section. The third function is simply to provide the reader with a knowledgeable background for the topics to be covered in the final portion of the chapter, where the techniques I have described will be seen in action.

The establishment of behavior: The first manipulative task faced by an experimenter is to get his subject to behave, to interact with the environment so that the experimenter can observe, record, and alter the nature of the interaction. With normal human subjects there is usually no problem in establishing behavior; the experimenter can use verbal instructions or other methods that take advantage of the subject's behavioral history. The task can be difficult, however, if the subject is a psychiatric or neurological patient, a retarded or preverbal child, or a lower animal.

Shaping: By applying the principle of reinforcement in an artful manner, the experimenter can shape the desired behavior out of the mass of responses available to his subject. Shaping is accomplished by reinforcing successively closer approximations to the behavior with which the experimenter ultimately wants to work. The experimental situation, for example, may be one in which a monkey is to be reinforced with food for pressing a lever. If the monkey just sits quietly at first, the experimenter will wait until the animal moves and will then immediately deliver the food. By continuing to reinforce all movements, the experimenter will soon have an active animal with which to work. He then reinforces only those responses which bring the animal closer to the lever. Within a few reinforcements, the monkey will have moved close to the lever, as if drawn by an invisible string. The experimenter now directs his attention to the animal's hand. He delivers the food whenever the hand moves closer to the lever, and it is not long before the animal places its hand on the lever and depresses it. The experimenter can then turn the rest of the job over to his automatic apparatus, which will deliver the food only when the animal actually depresses the lever. The shaping process is by no means species specific. It is applicable not only to a great variety of lower animals but also to humans who may range widely in intelligence, in the integrity of their nervous systems, or in the debilitating effects of psychiatric illness. Unless deliberate shaping of a patient's behavior has been attempted, it is unwise to conclude that he is unable to behave in a certain way. The process is particularly important in occupational therapy, where the establishment of behavior is a primary goal. We have much to learn about the shaping process, and a considerable amount of art is involved in shaping an organism's behavior, but there are a number of well-established practical rules that will help to ensure success:

1. Reinforce the behavior immediately. If the reinforcement is delayed, even by a fraction of a second, it is likely to be preceded by some behavior other than that which the experimenter intended to reinforce.
2. Do not give too many reinforcements for an approximation of the desired final response. Behavior that is initially reinforced must ultimately be extinguished as we move closer to the end point. If we reinforce intermediate forms of behavior too much,

these once-reinforced but now-to-be-discarded responses will continue to intrude and will unduly prolong the shaping process. There is, unfortunately, no quantitative method for predicting how many reinforcements are too many or, as we shall see below, how many are too few. The experimenter must take the subject's behavior as his guide, and if the subject tells him he has made a mistake he must be prepared to modify his own behavior accordingly.

3. Do not give too few reinforcements for an approximation of the desired final response. This is the most common difficulty in shaping behavior; the experimenter moves too fast. He abandons a response before he has reinforced it enough and, as a consequence, both the response and the variations which stem from it extinguish before he can mold the next closer approximation to the final behavior. The subject may then return to his original behavior, as if he had never gone through a shaping process at all. When this happens, the experimenter may be tempted to evade his responsibility by calling the subject stupid. What he must do is to start again and move the subject once more through the successive steps of the shaping process, taking care this time not to move too rapidly. If the experimenter is patient and willing to learn, he will usually find the subject equally willing.
4. Carefully specify the response to be reinforced in each successive step. Before abandoning one response and reinforcing the next approximation to the final behavior, the experimenter must watch the subject closely to determine what behavior is available for reinforcement. He should then specify that behavior as quantitatively as possible and adhere rigorously to the specification he has established. Otherwise he may inadvertently reinforce a slightly different but highly undesirable form of response and unnecessarily prolong the shaping process.

The maintenance of behavior: Reinforcement variables. Once the experimenter has established some behavior in his subject, he is faced with the problem of maintaining the behavior and keeping it available. A number of factors will influence his success in maintaining the subject's behavior: the state of deprivation of the subject; the type of reinforcement he uses; the size, or amount, of reinforcement; and the schedule that he follows in delivering reinforcements.

One of the first problems is satiation. If he has shaped the desired behavior with food reinforcement, for example, the experimenter can be certain that his subject will behave as usual in the experimental situation whenever he has been sufficiently deprived. Conversely, he can be certain that the subject will not behave as usual if he has been fully or partially satiated.

A problem related to satiation is the size of the reinforcements received by the subject. If these are too small, they will not maintain his behavior for any great length of time; if they are too large, the subject will quickly become satiated. The experimenter must find a useful compromise.

Food and other primary reinforcements are not always the most convenient types to use. Conditioned, or secondary, reinforcements may be more practical, particularly with human subjects. Environmental stimuli, not normally reinforcing in themselves, that control various segments of a subject's behavioral repertoire will eventually acquire a reinforcing function. For example, if a monkey is reinforced whenever a buzzer is sounding, we can then use the buzzer as a reinforcement to shape and maintain some other behavior in the animal. But just as food is a reinforcer only to an organism that has been deprived of food, a conditioned reinforcer that has been established through its control over food-reinforced behavior will be relatively ineffective unless the organism is food deprived. If there were no way around it, this dependence of a reinforcer upon a specific state of deprivation in the organism would severely limit the utility of behavioral control through reinforcement.

Fortunately both for laboratory investigation and for the richness of life outside the laboratory, conditioned reinforcers do not have to be so limited. A given stimulus can set the occasion for varied kinds of reinforcements: money, for example, and stimuli arising from the social environment, verbal stimuli, and others provided by friends, family, or institutional sources. Such stimuli have been termed "generalized reinforcers", for they are effective in a wide variety of environmental contexts and under a wide variety of deprivation states. Money will be an effective reinforcer at almost any time because a person is likely to be in at least one of the many deprivation states with which it is associated.

Even in the animal laboratory, when the experimenter begins to work with a new species of organism one of the major initial problems he will face is the selection of an adequate reinforcer. Standard food reinforcers are now available for rat, monkey, chimpanzee, and pigeon, but the problem has not yet been solved adequately for cat and guinea pig, for example. When the experimenter moves to human subjects the problem becomes even more acute, for he does not usually have sufficient control over the subject's state of deprivation to make food reinforcement practical. He must find other reinforcing agents that will still be powerful enough to generate and maintain stable behavioral patterns. When humans fail to replicate the orderliness of behavior shown by lower animals, the reason is often an inadequate reinforcer.

Long, Hammack, May and Campbell, using trinkets as reinforcers for children, found a deterioration in the orderliness of their subjects' behavior after several sessions of experimentation. Since the altered performance was similiar to that of lower animals which had become satiated after insufficient deprivation, Long and his co workers substituted new trinkets, thereby ameliorating the deteriorated performance. Stoddard (unpublished data), using candy reinforcement with children, observed similar changes, and was able to reverse them by varying the nature of the reinforcements within each experimental session, the children receiving candy, pennies, any of a wide variety of trinkets, or tokens that could be exchanged later for more valuable toys.

Ultimately, exchangeable tokens are probably the most feasible solution. If the experimenter cannot achieve adequate control over deprivation conditions, he should turn completely in the other direction and make use of generalized reinforcers. By using tokens, which can be exchanged for a wide variety of reinforcers, he can take advantage of whatever deprivation is currently effective in his subject. Generalized reinforcers have been used to advantage by Stoddard, Sidman, and Brady, working with normal and with psychotic adults in a hospital setting. They set up what was essentially a variety store, in which the subjects could trade their tokens for such objects as cigarettes, candy, magazines, books, records, art pictures, pipes, clothing, gift items, and many others. They could also trade their tokens for commercial trading stamps, which they could save and then trade for any of the items in the catalogue of the trading stamp company. Many of the subjects in this study came into the experimental cubicle almost daily, and performed in a consistently lawful fashion over a period of three years.

Morse and Dews (unpublished data), working with a prison population, have found that cigarettes are an effective generalized reinforcer in such an environment. The prisoners use them as a medium of exchange among themselves, and in this instance the experimenters do not have to maintain a supply of exchangeable items.

Bijou and Sturges, in reviewing some of the ways reinforcers have been used in studies with children, have pointed out that interactions between subject and experimenter can markedly alter the degree of control exercised by an ostensible reinforcer. The child brings with him into the laboratory a history of social interaction, and socially mediated factors such as signs of approval or expectation from the experimenter may override the effects of reinforcers like candy or trinkets. For example, a child may be spacing his responses in a manner appropriate to a temporal conditioning procedure with candy as reinforcement; but if the experimenter has also indicated his approval of the child's performance, the same behavior may continue even after the procedure has changed to one in which spaced responding is no longer efficient. The reinforcement from the experimenter may be more powerful than the candy, and the child's behavior may not come entirely under the control of the candy reinforcement. Bijou and Sturges suggest that human subjects be given minimal instructions, that all reinforcers be presented by mechanical or electronic means, and that the experimenter have as little contact with the subject as possible.

The point is well taken, but, as the writers themselves recognized, it may be difficult for the experimenter to isolate himself from the subject when the experiment itself is concerned with social interaction. Studies of verbal behavior, in which the reinforcement is also verbal, illustrate this difficulty very nicely. The effectiveness of any individual as a reinforcer will inevitably depend upon the subject's conditioning history.

It is possible, by appropriate instructions to the subject, to take advantage of types of conditioning history that are relatively consistent in the culture to which the subject belongs. We characterize the products of such conditioning histories with such common terms as competitiveness, self-respect, ambition, desire to please, etc. These terms are actually more descriptive of certain classes of generalized reinforcers than of any specific forms of behavior. The "signal detection" procedure devised by Holland has proven to be an extremely effective method for using a generalized reinforcer that is based upon instructions to the subject; the instructions, in turn, derive their effectiveness from an unspecified, but evidently general, set of cultural reinforcing practices.

Holland's subjects were asked to report whenever the pointer on a dial was deflected from its normal resting position. Their instructions were only to make as many detections as possible and to reset the pointer as rapidly as possible whenever a deflection was observed. At the end of each experimental session, the subject was told how many detections he had made and the average time taken per detection. This verbal interaction with the experimenter was sufficient to establish and maintain the pointer deflection as a reinforcer, and behavior was generated in the following way:

The subjects, working in the dark, could see the pointer only when they pressed a key that illuminated the face of the dial for a fraction of a second. When the subject observed that the pointer was deflected, he reported it by pressing another key, which reset the pointer. The deflections of the pointer were programmed so as to make possible various schedules of detections, or reinforcements. By recording the rate at which the subjects pressed the first button, thereby illuminating the dial, Holland was able to measure objectively the subjects' observing behavior.

Reinforcement schedules. In general, the greater the deprivation, the larger the reinforcement, and the more appropriate the type of reinforcement, the more successful we will be in keeping the subject behaving for long periods of time. Given adequate reinforcement variables, the schedule of reinforcement then becomes critical. I shall describe some of the more commonly used reinforcement schedules in order to illustrate the advantages and shortcomings of each, and to demonstrate the gross behavioral changes that may be brought about by some rather subtle alterations in the schedule of reinforcement. In these schedules the student of behavior has some powerful tools at his disposal, and he should be equipped to use them. I shall present only a few examples of published records for comparison with the known animal data, in order to provide some indication of the generality of the techniques.

1. Continuous reinforcement: The simplest technique is to reinforce the subject each time he responds appropriately. In one sense this is the most powerful technique, for it will keep the subject responding even when he is minimally deprived and when the size of each reinforcement is relatively small. But the continuous reinforcement schedule has at least one major disadvantage for experimentation; the subject is reinforced so frequently that he is likely to become satiated, making it impossible for the experimenter to observe his behavior over any substantial period of time.

Fortunately, we need not reinforce the subject for every response in order to maintain his behavior. Occasional reinforcements may maintain the response even more effectively than if we reinforced it every time. In fact, if we want to extinguish a subject's behavior, we must be absolutely consistent in withholding reinforcement. But, it should be noted, although we can maintain a subject's behavior by reinforcing only intermittently, we must then pay even more attention to deprivation and amount of reinforcement. Deprivation, reinforcement size, and reinforcement frequency are interlocking variables, and we must compensate for any decrease in one of these by increasing the others.

2. Fixed-interval reinforcement: One method of arranging reinforcements intermittently is to make them available to the subject only after a fixed period of time has elapsed; at the end of this period, the subject's next response will produce a reinforcement and the time interval will start again. If the experimenter has been able to secure an optimal arrangement of the important contributory variables the subject will adjust his behavior to the schedule in the manner shown in Figure. 3.1.

Holland has reported fixed-interval data obtained from Navy enlisted men. These subjects pressed a key which illuminated a dial, and the reinforcement for key pressing was a deflection of the needle on the dial. Figure 3.1 is a set of cumulative records from one subject for whom dial deflections were scheduled to occur, in different sessions, at fixed intervals of 1, 2, 3, and 4 minutes. The curves are very similar to those reported for lower animals. Each reinforcement is followed by a pause, the length of which is related to the duration of the fixed interval; as time elapses, the subject begins to respond and reaches a high rate before the next reinforcement. Curves for extinction after fixed-interval reinforcement also confirmed the animal data.

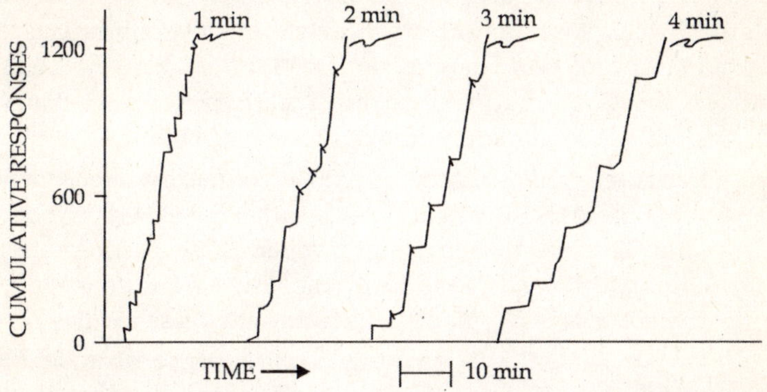

Fig. 3.1. Cumulative Records of One Subject's Observing Behavior when Reinforced on Fixed-interval Schedules of 1, 2, 3, and 4 Minutes.

Working with children four to eight years of age, who received trinkets, pennies, or projected pictures as reinforcement for pulling a lever or pressing a key, Long and his associates replicated some of the usual features of fixed-interval behavior, but were not able to maintain consistent performances on this schedule.

Stoddard, Sidman and Brady have also obtained fixed interval data that differs from the animal data usually reported. Their subjects were military personnel, both attendants and staff members, employed in a closed psychiatric ward in a military hospital. Generalized token reinforcers were used to maintain the subjects' lever pulling behavior. The subjects behaved very efficiently on the fixed interval schedule, pausing almost the full duration of each interval and then responding once or twice to procure the token almost on time. Many of the subjects used watches, however, and it is possible that if their behavior of looking at the watches could have been recorded, this would have yielded a typical fixed-interval picture, as did Holland's subjects when their observing behavior was recorded. When the experimenters placed an upper limit on the fixed interval, so that the subjects would miss an opportunity for reinforcement if they delayed their response as little as 0.5 second after the end of the interval, the records took on an appearance more like the expected one.

In general, the indications have been that the fixed-interval schedule is the least stable of all the reinforcement schedules in controlling human behavior. In animal work, too, however, fixed-interval behavior is notoriously sensitive to other variables, such as deprivation, reinforcement size, and novel stimuli. Holland's work suggests that stable and species-consistent fixed-interval behavior can be obtained in humans with appropriate techniques.

3. **Variable-interval reinforcement:** We can make reinforcements available to the subject at variable rather than fixed periods of time. The irregular spacing of reinforcements in time will eliminate the cyclic changes in response rate that characterize the subject's performance on a fixed-interval schedule.

If the variable-interval schedule is efficiently constructed, the subject will respond at a steady rate. The performance will be sensitive to the effects of many experimental operations, and because of its stability it will pose fewer measurement problems for the experimenter.

Figure 3.2 shows records obtained by Lindsley from six normal adult subjects who were reinforced with nickels on a one-minute variable-interval schedule. The response was lever pulling. Although there are wide individual differences in response rate, each individual's rate is steady and, although not shown here, is relatively consistent during many successive experimental periods. The curves resemble the animal data very closely. Holland, too, reports similar consistent response rates when the observing responses of his subjects are reinforced on a variable-interval schedule and, in addition, presents a more quantitative replication of the animal work. The response rates of his subjects decrease as the average interval of the variable-interval schedule is increased from fifteen seconds to two minutes.

The performance by children on variable-interval schedules in the experiments of Long, Hammack, May and Campbell also closely resembles that of other organisms. These investigators, however, noted that the construction of the variable-interval program was an important factor in determining the regularity of the children's performance. If there were too few short intervals in the program, there was considerable pausing and the records were generally irregular. This is to be expected, since too few short intervals will make the program more like fixed interval and will tend to generate a fixed interval performance; experimenters working with lower animals have also noted this phenomenon.

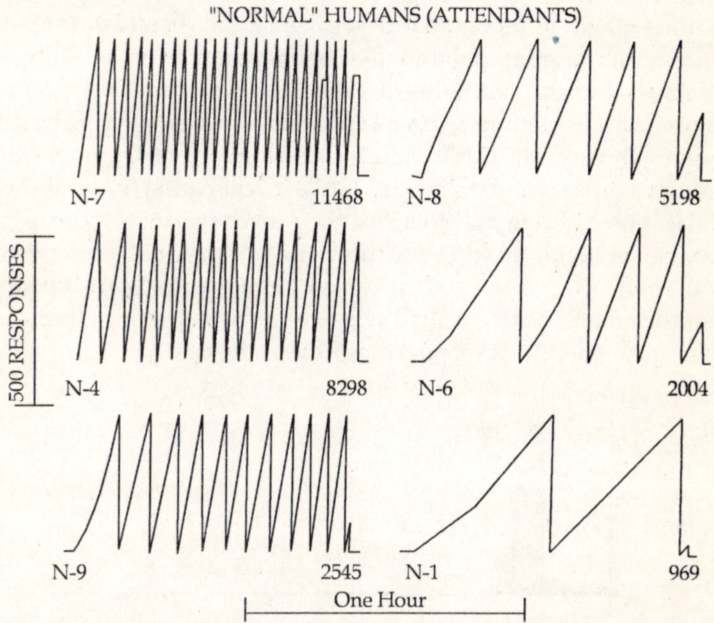

Fig. 3.2. Cumulative Records of the Behavior of Six Subjects Reinforced with Nickels on a Variable-interval Schedule.

4. Differential reinforcement of low rates: Reinforcement availability can be programmed simultaneously by a fixed-interval timer and by the subject's own behavior. For example, the timer may make reinforcement available every ten seconds, but only if the subject has not responded for ten seconds. Each response of the subject resets the timer and starts the ten-second period all over again. Every time the subject waits for ten seconds without responding, he will produce a reinforcement with his next response. Since responses that occur at a rate higher than one per ten seconds are extinguished, the schedule is characterized as the differential reinforcement of low rates, often abbreviated DRL. The resulting behavior is sometimes called timing behavior, or delayed response, for the subject must be able to delay his response for a specified period of time if he is to procure reinforcements.

Even with animal subjects, the DRL schedule can produce an empathic feeling of intense and painful concentration in the human observer. Experimenters who have themselves worked on this schedule report that it is extremely difficult for them to refrain from responding until the required time interval is judged to have elapsed. Nonetheless, the DRL schedule has proved extremely effective in maintaining stable and efficient behavior in human subjects. The frequency distributions of Figure 3.3 are from two of the children in Stoddard's investigation (unpublished data). The children had to space their lever-pulling responses at least ten seconds apart to procure candy; if they pulled the lever too soon, the ten-second interval began anew without any reinforcement; if they waited ten seconds or more since their last lever pull, their next response produced the candy.

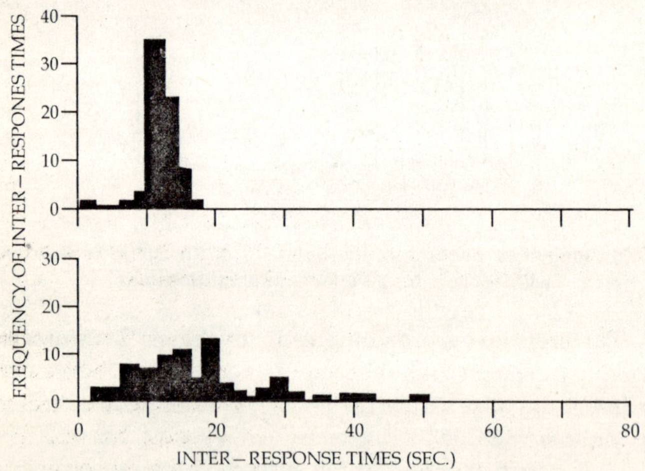

Fig. 3.3. Frequency Distributions of Interresponse Times, Obtained from Two Children Reinforced with Candy on a DRL Schedule. The Upper Record is from a Ten-year-old Child, the Lower from a 2.5-year-old.

The schedule was effective in generating low response rates in children ranging in age from 2.5 to 12 years. The older children were more precise in timing their responses, producing interresponse-time distributions with much less variability than is usually found with rats, but which are comparable with the performance of monkeys.

When the DRL schedule was shifted from ten to twenty seconds, the children decreased their response rates, and the interresponse-time distributions shifted appropriately. Also, many of the children were observed to go through a "superstitious" chain of responses between each lever pull; such behavior has also been reported with lower animals.

Holland found similar orderliness when his subjects' observing behavior was reinforced according to a DRL schedule that required them to pause at least thirty seconds between each observing response. He also confirmed an additional detail of the DRL performance that has been reported in several animal studies; when the subject responded just a little sooner than the required interval he often emitted a short burst of responses at a rapid rate.

Lane combined the Holland technique with the DRL schedule, but required a vocal utterance, the sound, "oo," as the observing response. His subjects were male and female undergraduates. Like animal subjects, they produced low response rates that were close to the value that would maximize the frequency of reinforcement. He also found appropriate shifts in response rate when he altered the length of the required pause.

Dews and Morse used a more complex version of the DRL schedule with male medical students who were reinforced with four nickels for pressing a telegraph key. Some subjects had to space their responses 2.5 seconds apart, and received their coins every hundredth time they did this; other subjects had to space their responses 25 seconds apart and were reinforced every tenth time they did so. The subjects were informed of the schedule. They were extremely efficient in spacing their responses; again the inter response-time distributions were more like those of monkeys than of rats. Dews and Morse also gave their subjects amphetamine, and the results were again consistent with those obtained from lower animals; the interresponse-time distributions were shifted in the direction of shorter interresponse times.

5. Fixed-ratio reinforcement: If we require the subject to respond a fixed number of times for each reinforcement, the availability of reinforcement will depend solely upon his own behavior. When we establish a fixed ratio of responses to reinforcements, the subject will behave as is shown in Figure 3.4; if he does not respond at a near maximal rate he does not respond at all. The pauses, when they occur, usually come just after a reinforcement.

In the investigations of Long and his coworkers, the children were also exposed to fixed-ratio schedules. Figure 4 illustrates two performances that confirm the findings from lower animals. In record 1, the subject had to respond 60 times for each reinforcement; in record 2, the ratio was shifted to 90 responses per reinforcement. These investigators also observed deteriorative changes similar to those previously described for the fixed-ratio behavior of lower organisms when the ratio size was increased too rapidly or when the subjects had accumulated large numbers of reinforcements.

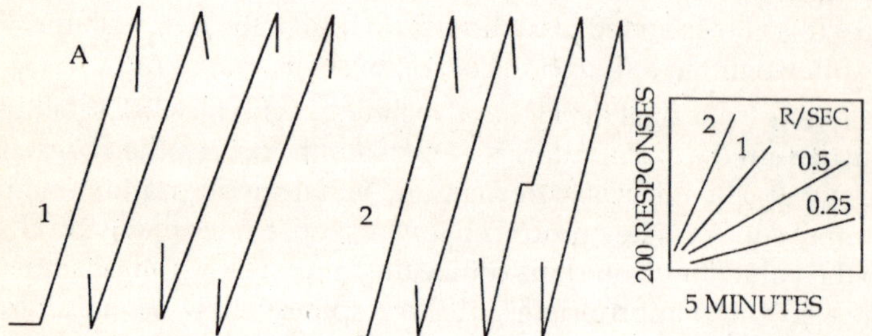

Fig. 3.4. Cumulative Records of the Behavior of a Child Reinforced on Fixed-ratio Schedule of 60 (record 1) and 90 (record 2) Responses Per Reinforcement.

Holland in his investigations of observing behavior in humans, also observed fixed-ratio performances characteristic of those obtained from lower animals with conventional reinforcement. And when he extinguished the observing response of his subjects, their extinction behavior exhibited the same special characteristics that are normally seen in the extinction records of animals after fixed ratio reinforcement.

6. Variable-ratio reinforcement: We can also make reinforcements available to the subject after variable rather than fixed numbers of responses. This schedule will generate the highest response rates of any described, and if the schedule is efficiently constructed the subject will hardly pause in his responding at all, even after receiving a reinforcement.

Variable-ratio schedules have not been used frequently with human subjects. Orlando and Bijou are the only investigators who have reported on this schedule and their work was with developmentally retarded children. Like infrahuman subjects, these retarded children responded at high steady rates on the variable-ratio schedule, with pauses being infrequent and not obviously related to the receipt of reinforcement.

Making behavior available: For reasons both of experimental convenience and control, the experimenter builds into his subject the behavior he wishes to investigate. First he shapes the behavior and then sets up the conditions to maintain it for the duration of the observation period. When he places the subject in the experimental situation, the desired behavior will appear.

But if the clinician is impatient, so is the experimenter, in his own way. He is not satisfied to have a single sample of behavior with which to work but wants to push on to greater complexity, to build several types of behavior into his experimental organism and study them all. There is the problem, then, of establishing a complex behavioral repertoire in a subject and subsequently making each component of the repertoire available for individual observation at the experimenter's convenience.

Stimulus control: An organism's behavior is governed not only by its reinforcing consequences but by the current environmental stimuli as well. This is vividly illustrated by the phenomenon of stimulus generalization. A pigeon, for example, is first reinforced on a variable interval schedule for pecking a disk that is illuminated with a particular wavelength of light. Then, during extinction, the illumination on the disk is changed periodically so that the bird is exposed to a number of other wavelengths in addition to the one that was present during reinforcement. The pigeon's rate of pecking will decrease as the stimulus differs more and more from the original one. The more the subject's environment changes, the less likely it is to behave in its usual fashion.

We can make deliberate use of environmental stimulus control to bring out the various components of a subject's built-in behavioral repertoire. When shaping the response and setting up the various conditions for its maintenance, we simply change some aspect of the environment to correspond with each of the separate maintenance conditions. For example, we may sound a tone while the subject is working on a fixed-interval schedule; when the subject is working on a fixed-ratio schedule we change the tone to a buzzer; and when the subject is avoiding shock we replace the auditory stimuli with a light. Eventually each of these stimuli will come to control its own form of behavior; whenever we turn on one of the stimuli the subject will respond appropriately to the experimental conditions correlated with the particular stimulus. The behavior is "on call," so to speak, at the experimenter's command.

It appears quite feasible to build more than one sample of behavior into the human subject and to place each form of behavior under stimulus control. Stoddard, Sidman, and Brady set up a multiple schedule with fixed-interval and fixed-ratio components; when a green light was turned on above the lever, the subjects were reinforced on a one-minute fixed-interval schedule, and when a red light was on, the reinforcement schedule was a fixed ratio of 50 responses per reinforcement. The schedule changed each time the subject received a reinforcement. Later, an upper limit was placed on the fixed interval, so that the subjects had to respond within 0.5 second after the end of each interval or else miss the reinforcement. Figure 5 illustrates the precision of the control exercised by the stimuli over the interval and ratio patterns of behavior. When the red light came on, the subject responded rapidly until he received a reinforcement and the light changed to green. With the onset of the green light, the subject paused for a while and then responded rapidly until reinforced. Both samples of behavior were thus available for observation in close temporal juxtaposition, and the effect of other variables could be assessed on each. Multiple stimulus control of fixed-interval and fixed-ratio behavior in the signal detection situation has also been shown by Holland to be of comparable precision.

With children as subjects, Stoddard (unpublished data) used a multiple schedule with variable-interval and DRL components. Competing effects from the subjects' reinforcement histories and a decline in the reinforcing power of the candies used as reinforcement in this study prevented good schedule control in some of the subjects, but where the schedule control was adequate, control by the corresponding stimuli was also precise.

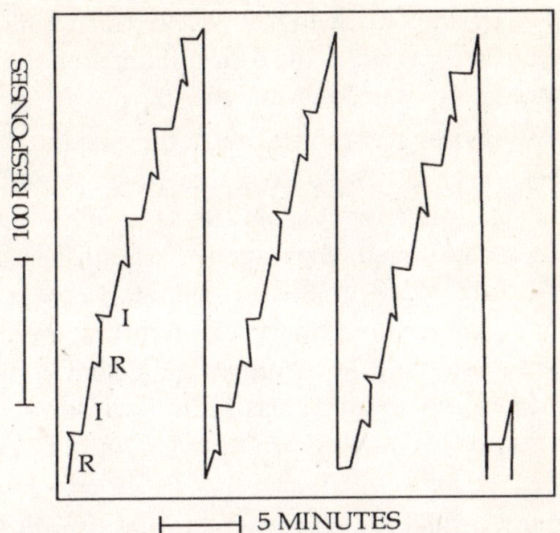

Fig. 3.5. Cumulative Records of One Subject's Behavior on a Multiple Fixed-interval, Fixed-ratio Schedule. The Pen is Deflected Downward During the Fixed-ratio Schedule. The Schedule Changed after each Reinforcement. The First Two Interval Segments are Indicated by the Letter I, and the First Two Ratio Segments by R.

Behavioral control through aversive stimuli: Aversive stimuli will reinforce, not the behavior by which the organism produces them, but rather the behavior which permits the subject to escape from them, or to terminate them. The most common stimulus of this type in the laboratory is electric shock, but others such as bright lights, loud noises, and excessive cold have also been used.

Conditioned suppression: The initial effect of a strong electric shock is to produce a general cessation of an animal's ongoing behavior. This disrupting effect of shock can, however, be placed under stimulus control. For example, we may first shape a monkey's lever-pressing response with food reinforcement and maintain the behavior with a variable-interval schedule. Then we shock the animal every ten minutes, but before each shock we turn on a tone for five minutes. The shock at first disrupts the monkey's lever-pressing behavior, but the disruption soon becomes channeled into the periods during which the tone is sounding; during these periods the animal ceases pressing the lever but returns to its normal performance after the shock. We now have available a technique for studying both the contributory and therapeutic effects of other variables upon a well-controlled behavioral disruption, a technique that will be particularly valuable if this phenomenon does indeed have relevance to "anxiety," a term that is frequently applied to it.

Escape behavior: Aversive stimuli may be used not only to suppress behavior but also to generate and maintain new responses. The simplest way to do this is to allow the subject to terminate, or escape from, the aversive stimulus whenever it is administered. Like food-reinforced behavior, escape-reinforced behavior can be maintained by various reinforcement schedules. The subject may succeed in turning off the shock only after the lapse of fixed or variable intervals of time (interval schedules), or after he has responded a fixed or variable number of times (ratio schedules).

Experimenters have been understandably reluctant to use electric shock with human subjects, and a number of other aversive stimuli have demonstrated their utility in a variety of experimental situations. Azrin, for example, used periods of rest from strenuous work. He instructed subjects to turn a hand wheel against a friction clutch to the limit of their physical ability. When the subjects were reinforced by a two-minute rest period after every 85 revolutions of the hand wheel, they increased the rate at which they turned the wheel and actually performed 50 per cent more work than when the rest periods were given independently of their behavior.

Avoidance behavior: Another way for organisms to deal with aversive stimuli is to prevent their occurrence-to avoid them. To generate avoidance behavior, we simply administer brief shocks to the subject, on either a fixed or irregular temporal schedule, and arrange conditions so that the subject postpones the shock each time he presses a lever. By pressing frequently enough, he could successfully prevent any shocks from occurring. With this procedure, the subject will respond at a steady rate for long periods of time, with the response rate being an inverse function of the amount of time the shock is postponed by each lever press. This behavior, too, can be brought under stimulus control to form an element in the experimental organism's multiple behavioral repertoire.

Using shock as an aversive stimulus for medical students, Ader and Tatum generated avoidance behavior which closely resembled that obtained with lower species. The subjects were given brief periodic shocks unless they pressed a button; each time they pressed the button, shock was postponed for a fixed period of time. Some of the subjects simply left the experimental situation, an escape response that is not usually available to animal subjects, but of those who remained, the majority learned to press the button within the first session. These subjects not only responded at the stable rates characteristic of avoidance behavior under this procedure, but their response rates were also inversely related to the amount of time each response postponed the shock, as has been found in animal studies. The subjects had no instructions on how to deal with the shock.

Azrin, using military personnel as voluntary subjects, generated escape and avoidance behavior with intense noise as the aversive stimulus. His basic technique was the signal detection procedure of Holland, the subjects' button-pressing responses being reinforced by needle deflection on a three-minute fixed-interval schedule. This produced the usual type of fixed-interval behavior, the subjects pausing after each reinforcement and then responding more rapidly until the next signal detection.

Once the fixed-interval baseline had been established, Azrin turned on an intense noise, allowing the subject to terminate the noise for five seconds (escape) with each observing response, or to postpone the onset of noise for five seconds (avoidance) each time he pressed the button when the noise was off. When these aversive contingencies were programmed concurrently with the fixed-interval schedule of signal detection, the temporal pattern of the subjects' behavior changed markedly. Instead of pausing after each signal detection, they pressed the button often enough to prevent the onset of noise. Near the end of the fixed interval, the usual high fixed-interval rate emerged from this initial avoidance behavior. Azrin was thus able to demonstrate avoidance and fixed-interval behavior concurrently in human subjects, replicating earlier data in which shock was used in a similar fashion with rats.

Azrin was also able to place this behavior under multiple stimulus control, with the noise acting as both aversive and discriminative stimulus. He did this by alternating three-minute periods with and without noise.

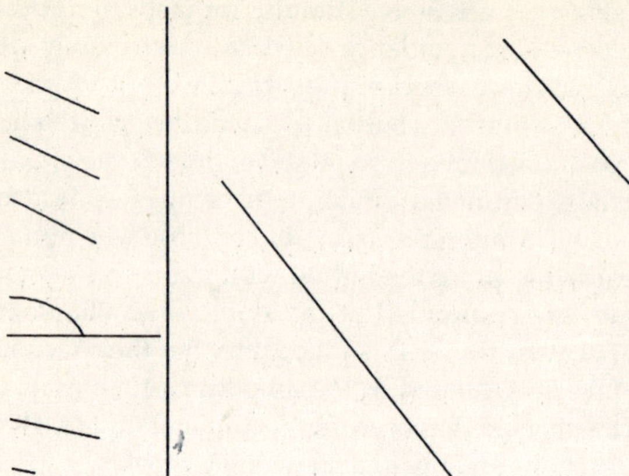

Fig. 3.6. Cumulative Records of Avoidance Behavior during the First Conditioning Session. The Oblique Markers Indicate Shocks. Shocks come at Different Frequencies (S-S) for each Subject, and each Subject Avoided Shock for a Different Period of Time (R-S).

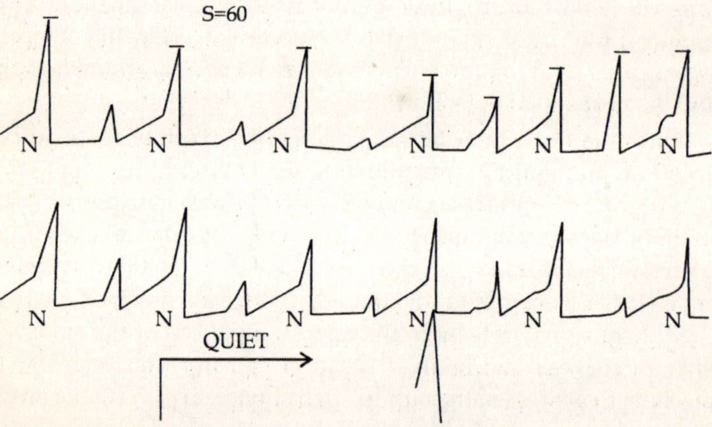

Fig. 3.7. Cumulative Records of a Subject's Performance when Reinforced by Signal Detection on a Three-minute Fixed-interval Schedule. In the Alternate Periods Marked N, each Response also Avoided an Intense Noise for Five Seconds.

Figure 3.7 shows some sample results; without noise, the subject displayed the typical fixed-interval performance, but when the noise was scheduled during alternate three-minute periods the records are typical of the concurrent fixed-interval and avoidance patterns.

This experiment is most encouraging with respect to the feasibility of extending to humans some of the techniques that have been developed in the animal laboratory for working with complex behavior.

Hefferline, Keenan and Harford have been able to condition an avoidance response that is so small as to occur unnoticed by the subjects, adult humans. A tiny twitch of the subject's left thumb, recorded electromyographically, served to terminate or to postpone noise that was superimposed upon music to which the subject was listening.

Lindsley used a pure tone to generate escape and avoidance behavior in an adult subject. Each time the subject closed a switch with his thumb, he reduced the intensity of the tone slightly. By operating the switch rapidly, the subject could quickly reduce the tone to zero intensity, and could then avoid the tone by continued responding. By operating the switch slowly, the subject could keep the tone at a moderate intensity. If the switch was not operated, the tone rose to and was maintained at its full intensity. Lindsley used this technique in a sleep-deprived subject to measure the duration and depth of sleep.

If animals are permitted to postpone the onset of a stimulus that is correlated with non reinforcement, or extinction, the response by which they can do so will be successfully conditioned and will display the usual characteristics of avoidance behavior. A similar technique has been used by Baer with preschool children. The children were permitted to watch cartoons, but occasionally the cartoons were interrupted. By pressing a lever, a child could reinstate the cartoon, and if he pressed the lever while the cartoon was still on he could postpone the next interruption. The technique of using a period of time-out from positive reinforcement as an aversive stimulus seems a promising one for human experimentation.

Basic Research Findings of Clinical Interest

Despite its emphasis on the resemblances between animal and human behavior in the laboratory, the preceding section was not intended to belittle the special problems of human behavior. My purpose was simply to demonstrate the applicability to human behavior of operant techniques that were developed in the animal laboratory. The evidence is more than merely suggestive.

Once it is known that the techniques are generalizable from subhuman to human, we can then place greater confidence in the generality of the findings that come out of these and related techniques. The following pages, therefore, will contain a selection-not by any means a thorough review-of some basic problems of clinical interest that have been raised, or even clarified, by the use of lower animals in the operant conditioning laboratory.

Stimulus generalization: Whenever an organism is reinforced or punished it is always in some environmental context, physical or social. The next time the organism encounters that same environment it will behave in the way for which it was previously reinforced, or in the same manner by which it was successful in dealing with the punishment; for example, by escape or avoidance. This may be considered a somewhat loose statement of a general behavioral principle. My concern here is with a related principle: the organism will also behave similarly when it encounters a situation that differs in some respects from the original one. This, again loosely stated, is the principle of stimulus generalization.

When a laboratory-derived behavioral phenomenon catches the attention of the clinical investigator or theoretician, he is rarely interested in those quantitative aspects of the data which are so dear to the experimenter's heart. He uses the experimental findings only in a qualitative way; the phenomenon is or is not relevant to a particular clinical problem. Stimulus generalization is an exception to this custom. Some of its most interesting and controversial extrapolations to clinical problems are based upon a quantitative assumption about the nature of the generalization gradient: namely, that behavior controlled by punishment will generalize in a quantitatively different manner, either more or less widely, than behavior controlled by positive reinforcement. Miller, for example, has based an ingenious theory of displacement on the assumption that the avoidance gradient is steeper than the approach gradient. Although no other theory has been stated as quantitatively as Miller's, the opposite assumption, that avoidance behavior generalizes more widely than approach behavior, is often invoked implicitly to explain the occurrence of phobias and other types of neurotic anxiety.

A most convincing demonstration that the latter assumption is correct has been provided by Hearst, who obtained simultaneous generalization gradients for punishment-controlled and reward-controlled behavior in individual monkeys. There were two responses available to the monkey concurrently; each time it pressed a lever it postponed shock for ten seconds, and when it pulled a chain it was occasionally rewarded with food on a variable-interval schedule. During subsequent generalization testing, both shock and food reward were discontinued, and the intensity of the cage illumination was systematically varied. The animal's rate of lever pressing (the avoidance response) did not change, regardless of how much the cage illumination varied from its original level. It pulled the chain (food reinforced response) progressively less frequently, however, as the cage illumination differed more and more from its original intensity. The avoidance gradient was flat and the reward gradient was relatively steep, with both gradients being measured simultaneously in the same animal.

The effectiveness of punishment in eliminating behavior: Punishment is a prevalent method of behavioral control in most cultural groups. Yet its role in the etiology of behavior disorders is a hotly debated issue, as is its utility in therapeutic techniques. Operant conditioning studies, however, as far as they have gone in this area thus far, yield a relatively clear picture of the effects of punishment. It is well established that the immediate consequence of punishment is to stop the organism from performing the punished behavior. There are also certain nonspecific effects of punishment: other responses than the punished one will also decrease in probability, a phenomenon that has been studied extensively by means of the conditioned-suppression technique: the effects of punishment will generalize to other situations than the one in which the organism was initially punished-stimulus generalization; if it is possible for the organism to avoid the punishment it will develop the behavior that permits it to do so, thereby, perhaps, substituting an even more undesirable response for the one that was initially punished.

But what are the long-term consequences of punishment with respect to the punished behavior itself? By using punishment, can we actually eliminate a response permanently from a subject's repertoire of behavior?

Azrin, using pigeons as subjects and electric shock as the aversive stimulus, has shown that if the organism continues to be reinforced with food for the punished behavior it will eventually begin responding again. The initial suppression of the punished response does not last. This is so even when the organism is shocked every time it responds and the food reinforcement is delivered only intermittently. Only when the shock intensity is extremely high will there be some permanent reduction in the animal's rate of response. Such high intensities, of course, are also most likely to generate the undesirable side effects of punishment, thereby increasing the cost at which we purchase the elimination of a particular response. Azrin also noted that when the shock is discontinued, the animal will respond for a while at a much higher rate than it ever did before being punished.

Even when other sources of reinforcement are eliminated, and the animal receives only punishment for its response, the initial suppression of the punished behavior is not likely to be permanent. Estes shocked rats while extinguishing their previously food-reinforced lever-pressing behavior. After they had stopped pressing the lever, he discontinued the shock. Soon the animals began to respond again, even though there was still no food reinforcement.

Both Estes and Azrin report a number of other corroborative and additional findings. The conclusion would seem to be that punishment is not a very efficient method for permanently eliminating behavior except via certain side effects like generalized suppression or avoidance.

Adventitious reinforcement: The principle of reinforcement is so pervasive in the experimental control of behavior that we sometimes take it for granted and fail to give it the respect it deserves. The experimenter sometimes sets up a contingency between the response of an organism and a subsequent reinforcement and then proceeds blithely to assume that he need only consider the particular contingency he has established. But the action of reinforcement is automatic, and independent of the intentions of the experimenter. Any behavior, whether or not he observes and measures it, that precedes the delivery of a reinforcement to the organism will be affected by the reinforcement. There need be no causal correlation between response and reinforcement; even when reinforcement follows a response adventitiously it will have the same effect upon that response as if the connection were a necessary one.

Skinner first demonstrated this by delivering food to pigeons at regular intervals, regardless of what they were doing at the time. Because a bird was necessarily doing something when the reinforcement came, its current behavior was "caught" and became a stereotyped performance, even though no such specific performance was necessary to produce the food. Skinner called this a superstition, because the animal's behavior was being maintained by a reinforcement over which it actually had no control; just as the rituals of the rain maker are maintained by occasional rainfalls.

Since Skinner's original experiment, adventitious reinforcement has come to play an increasingly important role in experimentation not only as a technical problem that is often difficult to solve but also as the key to a number of phenomena that would otherwise be difficult to understand.

For example, we may want to set up a discrimination experiment in which the animal is to respond only when a light is on. We turn the light on, let us say, every two minutes, and reinforce the animal only when it responds in the presence of the light. But we observe that the animal also responds when the light is off; furthermore, its temporal pattern of responses is typical of fixed-interval behavior. This is not simply a breakdown of behavioral lawfulness, an instance of behavior being maintained without reinforcement. The light in this experiment is a conditioned reinforcer, and because the animal happened to respond just before the light came on, the response was reinforced adventitiously, and began to occur more frequently when the light was off. And because the light was presented on a fixed interval schedule of two minutes, the subject's adventitiously reinforced behavior assumed the appropriate temporal pattern. Such behavior can easily be eliminated by arranging that the light will never come on if the animal has just responded.

Morse and Skinner have demonstrated yet another way in which a stimulus can develop adventitious control over an organism's behavior. Their baseline procedure was a variable-interval reinforcement schedule, with pigeons as subjects. The experimental operation was simply to turn on a blue light for four minutes once every hour. The blue light eventually assumed some control over the subjects' behavior, even though the variable-interval schedule remained the same, whether the light was on or off. Some of the subjects, for example, increased their rate of responding when the light was on. This happened because of accidental correlations between the light and the variable-interval program of reinforcement. Sometimes the light happened to come on when the schedule provided several closely spaced reinforcements, so that there was an adventitious correlation between the light and a higher-than-usual frequency of reinforcements delivered to the subject. The principle of reinforcement respects such a correlation, regardless of its utility, or lack of it, for the organism.

Behavior may become controlled adventitiously by aversive stimuli, also. In an experiment in which monkeys could obtain food by pulling a chain and, concurrently, could avoid shocks by pressing a lever, Sidman has shown that the food-reinforced response became involved adventitiously in the avoidance contingency, even though the response actually had no connection with shock avoidance. Simple temporal juxtaposition of the animal's chain pull and lever press, with the subsequent avoidance of shock, was sufficient to establish a spurious but powerful connection between chain pulling and shock avoidance.

A subject's behavioral history may contribute to the likelihood of adventitious control. Herrnstein and Sidman, working with monkeys, first developed a conditioned suppression of the animals' food-reinforced lever-pressing behavior. Then they trained the animals to press the lever to avoid shock. When the animals were again exposed to the conditioned-suppression procedure, they reacted by increasing their rate of lever pressing-just the opposite of suppression. The key to this phenomenon is the history of avoidance behavior that had been built into the animals. Because of this history, they reacted to the shock as if they could avoid it; an unreal and ineffective mode of adaptation, to be sure, but appropriate to their reinforcement history.

From these and other experiments there emerges at least one trend. The more complex the experiment-the more responses, stimuli, and types of reinforcement that are involved, and the more extensive the organism's behavioral history-the greater will be the likelihood of adventitious control over the behavior. The moral is evident, for what experimental situation involves more of these complexities than do the ordinary life situations of the behaving human? Because adventitious control is, in one sense, unrealistic control, its existence may give an impression of disorderliness in behavior, but the disorder is only in our interpretation, not in the behavior itself.

More unified presentations of related material are to be found in other chapters of this book. Let us now turn to some areas in which the laboratory has made closer contact with the clinic. The work I shall discuss in the following sections is still, in one sense, basic, for it is largely untried clinically, and is even occasionally speculative. But it is at least one step removed from "the study of behavior for its own sake and ultimately, perhaps, also for clinical relevance," and is in the direction of the study of behavior for its immediate clinical relevance.

Classification, Diagnosis and Therapy

There are numerous pathways through which an organism's behavior may be influenced. Anatomical structure, nerve chemistry, endocrine function, environmental input-to mention but a few-may all play a role in maintaining the stability and adaptiveness of one's behavior, or in producing malfunction-behavioral pathology. Behavioral breakdown, therefore, may originate in any of the systems and processes that are relevant to the normal functioning of the organism.

But regardless of their starting point all behavioral pathologies must pass through a final common pathway. Whether the pathology springs from a person's malfunctioning nervous system or from an unusual conditioning history, we can observe it only in the way he responds to and deals with his environment, both physical and social. The final common pathway, then, comprises the set of behavioral processes that govern the relations of the organism to his environment.

Here, then, is where the analysis of behavioral pathology must make its beginning. We must first be able to classify the patient's behavior in a fashion that will permit us to identify the behavioral processes involved in his particular problem. Once a useful behavioral classification has evolved, we may then go on to seek other correlates that will help to define the disease process.

Our gross preliminary observations tell us little more than that the patient is not behaving as he should. Perhaps he finds himself involved in a paranoid plot; or walls himself off in autistic silence; or develops an aphasic inability to name objects. Such classifications-paranoia, autism, aphasia-are too general to form a maximally useful diagnostic base. Patients given one label are found to differ among themselves in the etiology of their breakdown, in their response to similar treatments, in their specific patterns of behavior. What is required is a set of general behavioral principles which will serve to regroup behavioral pathologies into classes that may be differentiated in terms of the behavioral processes involved.

For example, we may have a patient who cannot say nouns. Can this symptom be the basis for a class of neurological disease? What status do nouns have in the elucidation of behavioral processes? In themselves, they have no status at all. They are verbal responses, and as such may participate in many different behavioral processes. We may hold up a pencil and ask the patient to tell us what it is, and he may be unable to name it. Yet if we ask him to write his name he may immediately say, "Give me a pencil." The response, pencil, is under two different forms of behavioral control in this example. One of these forms of control is defective; the other is intact. The case may be no different in principle from that of a rat which, after it has undergone an experimental brain lesion, will no longer press a lever if we give it food for doing so, but will continue pressing a lever that serves to avoid shocks. The animal's response is the same, but it is under two forms of environmental control; the brain lesion affected only one of these.

Approaches to Classification

Operant techniques and the principles derived from them have only just begun to be applied to problems of classification. The validity of the attempts has yet to be established, and perhaps it is even too soon to try this, for the range of phenomena that have been touched upon is still narrow and no single problem has yet been analyzed in depth. The approaches to classification may themselves be subdivided in terms of their methods of analysis.

The educated guess: This is a strictly clinical approach, in that it relies upon direct observation of the patient in a non experimental setting. As in the best clinical tradition, however, the observations are made against a background of existing knowledge. In the present instance, this background consists of laboratory-acquired knowledge of the processes by which a person's behavior is established and maintained. Ferster has given an excellent exposition of this approach, based upon Skinner's extensions of operant principles to problems of social interaction.

One begins simply by observing the patient's current behavior, analyzing his performances in terms of known behavioral processes, and then making guesses about the ways these processes might have been historically manipulated so as to produce the patient's particular difficulties. Ferster elaborates a number of ways of classifying the psychiatric patient in terms of such a functional analysis, with emphasis upon the role of the social environment.

For example, the patient may lack "parts of the complex repertoire necessary to achieve reinforcement from the complicated social environment". He may be deficient verbally, or unable to engage in everyday social intercourse. This could have come about through an inadequate reinforcement history. The behavior may simply not have been built into the person. If the behavior is not established at the appropriate time it may be very difficult to do so later. A child's initial approximations to socially desirable behavior will be accepted as part of the shaping process, but society demands greater precision from the adult and will not reinforce his "childish" approximations.

The person can actually possess the required behavior but fail to engage in it because the current reinforcement conditions are not optimal with respect to amount, frequency, or schedule. The behavior is available but cannot be maintained. Or excessive punishment may have generated avoidance behavior that successfully competes with more adaptive forms of response.

When behavioral classification is made by means of educated guesswork, its ultimate validation must come via therapeutic success. The therapist must actually manipulate the variables he suspects are relevant in any particular case. As Ferster points out:

If the therapist is ultimately to be successful, he must alter the relationship between the patient's performance in a wide variety of social situations and the reinforcement and punishment which will result. It is possible that many of the symptoms which bring the patient to therapy are largely a by-product of inadequate positively reinforced repertoires; that the disposition to engage in the psychotic, neurotic, and pathological behaviors may seem strong when compared to weak existing repertoires but would disappear as soon as alternative effective ways of dealing with some accessible environment are generated.

This is, indeed, an active conception of therapy. It is based upon the assumption that a patient's behavior, whatever historical factors may have been responsible for its present state, is manipulable through variations in the concurrent controlling environment. And, insofar as it is feasible, it extends therapeutic practice from the therapist's office out into the community of which the patient is a member, the community whose reinforcing practices will eventually pronounce judgment upon the success or failure of the therapy.

Ferster and DeMeyer have undertaken a detailed analysis of autistic children's performance and have described several kinds of historical circumstances which might have brought about their behavioral deficits. Based on his preliminary classification, which he stated in terms of a functional analysis of operant behavior rather than the usual diagnostic categories, Ferster made an intensive study of the practices which might be effective in developing a behavioral repertoire in the autistic child. In a controlled environment, he used the techniques of shaping, reinforcement schedules, stimulus control, extinction, conditioned reinforcement, and generalized reinforcement. Through these techniques, the children learned to manipulate various automatic devices, starting with a simple electrical switch for which they were reinforced with food. More complex performances were built up gradually, the children finally behaving with great accuracy on a matching-to-sample procedure. Various kinds of reinforcers were used: food, candy, music, an opportunity to play a pinball machine, a picture viewer, etc. Later, coins were established as generalized reinforcers, and the children could use these to operate devices that allowed them to watch cartoons, to get a trained animal to perform, to play with an electric organ, a motor-driven rocking horse, an electric train, or a television set, or to obtain a life jacket and go to the swimming pool. They also learned to save up coins and to use them only when appropriate stimuli indicated that the coins would be effective for "purchasing" something.

After considerable refinement of the techniques, the autistic children exhibited essentially normal behavior in the experimental environment for several hours at a time. Therapy, of course, was far from complete. Outside the controlled environment the children were still autistic, and even within the environment they still had not developed a repertoire of social behavior. It remains to be seen whether operant techniques can accomplish these extensions.

The educated guess has also received some experimental-therapeutic validation in a few other areas. Flanagan, Goldiamond and Azrin were able to control stuttering in chronic stutterers through operant techniques. They succeeded in increasing the frequency of stuttering by permitting the subject to turn off or to avoid a loud tone with each non fluency; conversely, they also decreased the frequency of stuttering by punishing each non fluency with the same loud tone. As they point out, stuttering is open to an operant analysis, and the direct operant control of stuttering may be a more profitable line of therapy than attempts to treat it as a by-product of "anxiety." Again, however, there is the problem of generalizing the therapeutic effect from the laboratory to the normal environment.

Ayllon and Michael, analyzing the ward behavior of hospitalized psychiatric patients, concluded that many of the problems these patients presented were the direct result of reinforcement in the hospital setting. They were concerned, not with the behavior that led to the patients' admission to the hospital, but rather with the annoying and disturbing behavior displayed by some patients in the hospital setting and which " may become so persistent that it engages the full energies of the nurses, and postpones, sometimes permanently, any effort on their part to deal with the so-called basic problem,"-such behavior as "failures to eat, dress, bathe, interact socially with other patients and walk without being led, hoarding various objects, hitting, pinching, spitting on other patients, constant attention-seeking actions with respect to the nurses, upsetting chairs in the dayroom, scraping paint from the walls, breaking windows, stuffing paper in the mouth and ears,". They instituted a specific program of operant control to reduce the frequency of such disruptive activities, with psychiatric nurses playing the role of "therapists."

By extinguishing the undesirable behavior, for example by refusing to give a patient attention when she habitually entered the nurses' office, or by not reacting in any way to a patient's delusional talk, the nurses were able to reduce the incidence of such behavior to the point where it was no longer troublesome to them in their routine duties. Another technique they used with a violent patient was to reinforce incompatible behavior. Escape and avoidance conditioning were used with two patients who consistently refused to eat unless aided by the nurses. Since both of these patients were extremely concerned with keeping their clothes neat and clean, the nurses instituted the practice of spilling some food on the patients' clothing whenever they insisted on being spoon fed. The patients could avoid this by feeding themselves. In both cases, the program ultimately resulted in complete self feeding by the patients.

Slack has applied operant shaping techniques to the problem of introducing hitherto unreachable adolescent delinquents to psychotherapy. By working with the boys not as patients but as experimental subjects, Slack created a situation in which he was able to pay them for participating in the project. But long before any therapeutic relationship could develop, the problem of maintaining reliable contact with the subjects had to be solved. Schwitzgebel has described the technique that was developed:

Following the initial contact, the boy may arrive at any time during the day. Whenever he arrives and for whatever reasons, his attendance is immediately reinforced by the sharing of food such as cokes, fruit, or sandwiches. Immediately after his talking into the recorder he is paid in cash. He may then help to build electronic equipment, listen to music, take driving lessons, or participate in other rewarding activities. When his hour or so is up, a time convenient for him is set for the next day. At first the experimenter is not particular about his early or late arrival. Only after attendance becomes dependable is there an attempt to get him to arrive on time. This is done by paying the boy more the nearer he arrives to the correct time or by using unexpected bonuses. Gradually, then, a time more convenient for the experimenter is set. Within 15 to 30 meetings the boys generally arrive very dependably, on time, and at the experimenter's convenience.

The shaping procedure has proved to be efficient in establishing consistent attendance. Subsequently, and at the subjects' own pace, the major source of reinforcement shifts from the salary to the interpersonal relationship that develops between experimenter and subject. The work is still in an early stage, but there are strong indications that once the initial hostility and suspicion are overcome the delinquent is as capable of accepting therapy as is the ordinary middle-class neurotic.

Laboratory testing for behavioral deficit: The educated guess provides, at best, a non quantitative classification of behavioral pathology. An autistic child, for example, may be a victim of a history of general non reinforcement; a delusional patient may be a product of too much reinforcement; stuttering may be an instance of reinforcement that has been inappropriately applied. These are all-or none classifications. This is not to deny their potential value, which is likely to be especially great in the hands of a practitioner who is familiar with operant principles and at the same time has considerable clinical experience. But the techniques of operant conditioning in the laboratory permit a precision of behavioral analysis far greater than the educated guess can provide. There have, therefore, been a number of attempts to correlate behavioral pathology with the patient's performance in relatively well-controlled laboratory settings.

Perhaps the most extensive program of this sort is one that was initiated by Lindsley, Skinner and Solomon with hospitalized chronic psychotics. Through long-term testing of the operant behavior of individual patients, they have been attempting to identify syndromes of behavioral deficit, in the hope that such syndromes would define subclasses of psychosis. In the basic technique, the subjects voluntarily enter a small room. The room contains a panel on one wall, and on the panel are located a plunger the patient can pull and a small aperture through which reinforcements can be delivered. Most of the data thus far have been obtained by reinforcing the patients with candy for pulling the plunger, the reinforcement schedule being a one-minute variable interval.

Approximately 15 per cent of the adult patients refused to enter the room, either initially or after a few days of testing. Shaping eventually brought in several of the most deteriorated members of this group. Only 10 per cent of the patients pulled the plunger at normal rates for this reinforcement schedule-above 800 responses per hour. The remaining 75 per cent of the patients responded at low, irregular rates, with frequent pauses. This initial success in achieving a gross differentiation between psychotic and normal populations, even with such a simple technique, encouraged the investigators to undertake a further analysis of the low response rates characteristic of the psychotic patients.

The first, and perhaps the most striking observation, was that each patient engaged in his characteristic psychotic symptom during the pauses in plunger pulling. "For example, the pacer paced, the hallucinator berated the empty room, the destructive patient tore his clothing, the compulsive patient made patterns out of his candies on the floor, the depressed patient just sat, etc". This observation suggests that psychotic processes function as competing response systems in the operant testing situation; that the frequency and duration of pauses in the patient's operant performance can be used as an index of the frequency and duration of discrete psychotic episodes or incidents.

Since inadequate reinforcers can also produce low and erratic response rates, the investigators explored a variety of reinforcers with a group of male chronic psychotics: candy, female nude pictures, male nude pictures, five-cent pieces, feeding a hungry kitten, and extinction (no reinforcement).

In general, candy emerged as the most effective reinforcer, but the most interesting data with respect to classification were the "motivation profiles" that were constructed for each individual patient. Examples of five such profiles may be seen in Figure 8 . Patient P10 responded only for candy; patient P32 responded for candy and for the generalized reinforcer, nickels; all of these patients responded at low rates for female nude pictures, but two of them, patients P20 and P35, responded at higher rates for male nudes- both of them had been observed engaging in homosexual practices within the hospital; patients P35 and P37 responded at high rates in extinction, when no reinforcement was being provided at all.

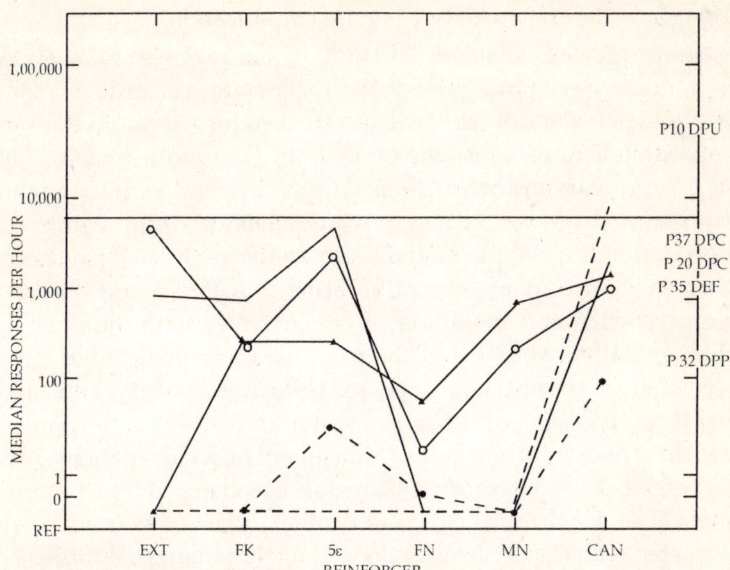

Fig. 3.8. Response Rates for Five Subjects when Working for Different Reinforcers. EXT, no Reinforcements; FK, Feeding a Kitten; 5¢, Nickels; FN, Female Nude pictures; MN, Male Nude Pictures; CAN, Candy.

Other types of profiles, too, were obtained from the group of patients tested. What we have here is the beginning of a behavioral subclassification, based upon the types of reinforcers that are effective for each individual. Some of the patients show a deficiency in the extent to which their behavior is controlled by generalized reinforcement (nickels), or by specific types of conditioned reinforcers (male or female nude pictures, or feeding a kitten), or by lack of reinforcement (extinction). None of these, by itself, is likely to define a class of psychosis that will be useful to the diagnostician or therapist; but when these profiles can be examined in combination with others for different variables, useful clusters are likely to emerge. The clusters may show little correlation with current schemes of psychiatric diagnosis, but such correlations should not be the goal of behavioral classification. A behavioral classification of behavioral deficit, based upon objective, manipulable variables, will single out those factors to which the therapist must give his attention; again, as with the educated guess, therapeutic success will be the final criterion of the effectiveness of such a classification.

Lindsley has extended the study of the variables relevant to psychotic behavior in a number of directions, and I can do no more than mention some of these. He has studied long-term rhythms in response rate of patients who came to the laboratory almost daily for several years and has correlated these rhythmic variations with psychiatric diagnosis, ratings of ward behavior, drug treatments, social variables, and physical disease. In the analysis of psychosis as a competing response system, vocal hallucinatory symptoms have been recorded and manipulated concurrently with the operant plunger-pulling behavior of the patients. Extensive studies have been made of patients who appeared to be insensitive to extinction; that is to say, who never stopped responding after reinforcement was discontinued. The mode of adjustment of several patients was studied when the reinforcement schedule was changed from variable interval to fixed ratio. Drugs and other types of therapy were evaluated with respect to their effects upon the patients' performance in the operant situation.

Extensive as these investigations have been, they are as yet only a beginning. They do little more than suggest that a purely behavioral classification of psychosis is possible, and indicate some of the lines an attempt at such classification may follow. More extensive sampling of the psychotic population is still required, not for statistical purposes but to ensure evaluation of all possible varieties of the illness; more extensive investigation of behavioral variables must be undertaken in order to ensure that all possible avenues of behavioral control are included in each patient's profile; and when a workable classification begins to emerge, therapeutic validation must be attempted.

Some initial applications of operant techniques to the problem of classification have been made with populations other than the chronic psychotic adult. Lindsley has demonstrated the applicability of the techniques to psychotic children. Orlando and Bijou have shown that simple and multiple reinforcement schedules can maintain the behavior of retarded children, and they suggest that these behavioral baselines are well suited to the study of discrimination, generalization, and motivation in such children.

Ellis, Barnett, and Pryer have made similar observations, even with retardates of a type usually labeled "untestable," and have, in addition, found a positive relation between response rates and mental age in retarded children. They also noted that the performance of severely defective children was characterized by frequent pauses, similar to those found in Lindsley with adult psychotics. This observation underscores the need for more detailed profiles for each patient; a single indicator may suggest pathology but is not likely to differentiate subclasses of pathology.

Laboratory testing of specific behavioral variables: Lindsley has pointed out that psychotics are not always psychotic: "Psychosis, defined in terms of the behavior that hospitalizes a person, is most often highly infrequent". Similarly, clinical neurologists are well aware that behavioral deficits or abnormalities are highly variable in a given patient, sometimes showing up in one examination and then being absent in an examination at a different time. Such observations require that we look more closely at the concept of "deficit." If the patient sometimes has a particular response or set of responses, and sometimes does not, in what is he deficient?

It is highly likely that the deficiency exists not in the patient's behavior but in some variable or set variables that controls the behavior. If we do not recognize the different variables that may control a given response, we may easily fail to recognize differences in our behavioral tests. In one situation we may try to elicit the behavior by applying the variable whose control is defective; in another situation we may apply a variable whose control is intact and the behavior may appear where it was previously absent. This is surprising to us only so long as we do not have an adequate classification of the relevant variables. A second type of laboratory test of operant behavior, then, will look not for behavioral deficit but for unusual functional relations between behavior and its controlling variables.

In his analysis of verbal behavior, Skinner has outlined a number of classes of relation that may exist between verbal responses and their controlling variables. Even though the form of a verbal response may be the same on different occasions, it cannot be treated as the same operant if it is determined by different factors. Hughlings Jackson made a rough distinction of a similar sort when he differentiated between two kinds of speech, emotional and propositional: patients with motor aphasia who were unable to say voluntarily more than a few words could nevertheless swear exceedingly well; or an aphasic who could say almost anything "by accident" could not say the same thing when he wished. Skinner's classification goes into considerably more detail, and only a brief summary can be given here of some of the types of functional relations he describes.

Take, for example, the vocal response, "water." One form of this response may be largely controlled by a person's state of water deprivation; if he is unable to emit the operant, "water," when thirsty, we may assume that the control of deprivation is deficient. A different type of control is involved when we show the person some water and ask him to name it. The naming of objects is largely under stimulus control, and the consequences of such behavior are often of more immediate benefit to the listener than to the speaker. A patient in whom the functional relation between deprivation and the response, water, is intact, may nevertheless show a deficiency in stimulus control and be unable to identify water on demand. Still other types of behavioral control are involved when a person is asked to echo the response, water, after it has been pronounced by someone else, or to read it aloud from a text. But because textual and echoic responses have usually been strongly conditioned-they are among the earliest forms of control established in the child-these functional relations may remain intact when at the same time the patient may be unable to fill in the blank in the statement, "The boat hit an iceberg and rapidly filled with -." The response in this instance is under the control of other verbal responses, and such intraverbal control, usually less strongly conditioned than textual or echoic control, may be deficient.

As Skinner points out, this "... is not a classification of forms of response, since we cannot tell from form alone into which class a response falls. In order to classify behavior effectively, we must know the circumstances under which it is emitted". There have as yet been no definitive tests of Skinner's classification of verbal behavior, but with the experimental material already at hand in the form of a large aphasic population, we may look forward to the increasing application of operant techniques and principles to the pathology of verbal behavior.

There has, however, been a small beginning made in a similar direction with respect to nonverbal operant behavior. Stoddard, Sidman, and Brady, working with acute psychotics in a military hospital, have been attempting to identify the lines along which behavioral control has fractured in these patients. The variable upon which they have concentrated thus far has been reinforcement frequency. They used a complex procedure consisting of the following elements: The subjects had two plungers available, and obtained token reinforcements for pulling one of them (the reinforced response). The basic token-reinforcement schedule was a multiple fixed interval, fixed ratio. When the subjects were working on the interval schedule, however, the length of the interval doubled after they received each token; similarly, when they were working on the ratio schedule, the number of times they had to respond to obtain a token doubled each time they received one. Thus, the reinforcement frequency on each schedule decreased whenever the subject obtained a token.

By pulling the second plunger (the switching response), the subject could change the schedule from interval to ratio or vice versa, and when the schedule changed, the progressively increasing sequence began anew at the lowest interval or ratio value. The likelihood that the subjects would switch from one schedule to the other was manipulated by placing the switching response on a ratio schedule. A fixed number of switching responses was therefore required before the subject could change the schedule and return the reinforcement frequency to its highest level.

When a large number of responses was required to switch the schedule, the subjects could maximize the reinforcement frequency by switching less often. For example, if the subject had to respond 88 times to change the schedule from fixed ratio to fixed interval, it would not be very efficient for him to switch when he could obtain the next token after only 11 responses. He could obtain more tokens in a shorter period of time if he postponed the changeover until the ratio schedule for the reinforced response was more nearly equal to the ratio schedule for the switching response. On the other hand, if only 11 responses were required to change the schedule, the subject could increase the frequency of reinforcement by switching more often.

The non hospitalized subjects and several of the patients were found to adjust their behavior in such a way that they maximized the frequency of reinforcement each time the switching requirement was increased. The behavior of several patients, however, was not under the control of reinforcement frequency; as the number of responses required to change the schedule increased, they failed to adjust their switching behavior in such a way as to keep reinforcement frequency at its highest possible level. Their efficiency curves, measured in terms of reinforcement frequency, declined as the switching requirement increased.

Here was a clear indication that a basic variable was not controlling the behavior of some of the patients in a manner consistent with normal behavioral control. Interestingly enough, these patients were assigned the least favorable psychiatric prognosis-arrived at independently of the experimental findings-at the end of their treatment period. But again, it is unreasonable to expect an adequate classification on the basis of one variable alone. We can anticipate not only that some patients will be controlled normally by reinforcement frequency but that some otherwise efficiently functioning people will exhibit abnormal control. Techniques will have to be developed for checking other basic variables, both singly and in interaction with each other, and any valid classification will have to be based upon complete profiles of behavioral control. Again, too, the classifications are not likely to conform closely to current psychiatric categories. The ultimate validating step will come from therapeutic attempts to restore the normal functional relations between a patient's behavior and those variables whose control has been found to be deficient.

4

Intelligence and Its Measurement

The important role played by the development of intelligence testing in stimulating the growth of the early psychological clinic. In the last chapter we talked about the value of having an estimate of a patient's intelligence when we are trying to do a thorough job of diagnosis. We are now prepared to look into the theoretical and practical side of the measurement of intelligence a little more carefully. The student who wishes to have a thorough grasp of this field will have to supplement his reading with one or more of the many source books and texts which cover the measurement of intellectual capacity.

The Nature of Intelligence

The beginning student will discover through his readings that there are many definitions of intelligence. This is apt to be perplexing to him. Most laymen are satisfied that they understand the meaning of the term. In our everyday conversation, we continually hear statements like, "He's not very bright," or "Any normally intelligent person can see," and so on. Our working ideas about intelligence seem to make sense, and so we may not worry about the technical problem of definition. However, there is considerable confusion among psychologists over the question of the definition and nature of intellectual capacity. Some disagreement exists over what is being measured and what should be measured by our well-established intelligence tests.

In our discussion of the historical development of testing, we said that the measurement of intelligence did not become popular until emphasis had shifted from the simple reaction-time and sensory-motor tests of Galton to the complex types of tasks of Binet. Galton and Cattell, who were theoretically oriented, believed that their tests measured the basic units of mental capacity. On the other hand, Binet faced the practical problem of differentiating between defective children and those who were lazy. As we have seen, it eventually became apparent that the sensory-motor tests would not do what was expected of them, i.e., correlate well with academic success. However, the Binet type of test proved immediately useful; and while Binet 's procedures did not take hold in this country right away, they eventually became the core of the great testing movement later on. The Binet tests were useful because they succeeded in differentiating between children of various age and grade levels and made possible the prediction of the child's progress in school.

Though Binet 's theoretical approach was vague and not formally worked out, it was a global one. He assumed that intelligence was a single general attribute. Most of the people who measured intellectual capacity after Binet were clinicians. They were interested in measures that worked because they were dealing with children or adults in the clinic or school system. The global concept of intelligence seemed to be successful and became firmly established in the succeeding years.

Definitions: Let us look at some of the definitions of intelligence that have been proposed. Freeman classifies these definitions into four types. The first places its emphasis on the adjustment or adaptation of the person to his total environment or aspects of it. In 1914, for example, Stern wrote, "Intelligence is a general capacity of the individual consciously to adjust his thinking to new requirements."

The second type of definition discussed by Freeman stresses learning ability as the important feature in intelligence. The idea of intelligence being characterized by learning ability or related to it has interested a number of investigators. The problem is complicated by the fact that intelligence scores are not really independent of learning. Nevertheless investigators have correlated rate of learning with intelligence test scores. In virtually all these studies the relationship has been positive. Depending upon the type of material to be learned, the correlations range from 0 to.80. Multiple correlations between intelligence and several learning tasks tend to be higher than the single-order correlations. This sort of work has allowed us to say that, depending upon the material, a positive relationship exists between intelligence and ability to learn. What the true relationships are we cannot legitimately say because of the extreme range of correlations found.

A third type of definition of intelligence has stressed the ability to carry on abstract thinking. Terman 's definition is a good example of this kind of concept. He writes, "An individual is intelligent in proportion as he is able to carry on abstract thinking." In this connection it is interesting to note that studies comparing intelligence test scores with problem-solving tasks which involve abstract relations, reasoning tasks, and inference situations have correlated little better, on the whole, with intelligence than the simple learning of verbal material and perceptual-motor skills. Our current intelligence tests stress abstract concepts of intelligence.

Finally, there is a class of definitions that attempts to be broader in scope than any of the foregoing ones. These definitions are more comprehensive in the sense that they combine and enlarge the other three types of definitions.

For example, Wechsler states that "intelligence is the aggregate or global capacity of the individual to act purposefully, to think rationally and to deal effectively with his environment." Stoddard maintains that "intelligence is the ability to undertake activities that are characterized by (1) difficulty, (2) complexity, (3) abstractness, (4) economy, (5) adaptiveness to a goal, (6) social value, (7) the emergence of originals, and to maintain such activities under conditions that demand a concentration of energy and a resistance to emotional forces."

In examining this sample of definitions which have been published by well-known psychological scholars, several questions arise. In the first place it is clear that the tests we have available do not measure all the aspects that have been attributed to intelligence by these definitions. It has been pointed out again and again by clinicians like Doll, Sarason, Jastak and others that two feeble-minded children with the same score on the Stanford-Binet may behave quite differently with regard to social effectiveness. It is not always possible to decide whether these children should be institutionalized on the basis of the IQ alone. Therefore, the section in Wechsler 's definition of intelligence which deals with ability to "deal effectively with his environment" does not apply to the measurements derived from our most useful intelligence tests. This example of the void between definitions of intelligence and its actual measurement can be multiplied many times.

How, then, do most of the definitions of intelligence come into being? In part they are based on a collection of armchair ideas resulting from the observations of people inside and out of the psychological clinic. They also arise from inspection of what intelligence test scores actually predict. In any case they do not really define the nature of the mental organization. They more or less identify what the intelligent person can and cannot do with a variety of problem situations. The definitions are logical and descriptive statements which are often stated in such a way that it is difficult to have any idea of how the kind of intelligence specified can be measured. Examine the definition given by Munn in his introductory textbook on psychology. He writes, "Intelligence is flexibility or versatility in the use of symbolic processes." But what Munn means by the words flexibility and versatility is not made very clear.

When we examine the definitions of intelligence discussed above, we notice that they assume that intelligence is some kind of general attribute more or less of which exists in everyone and which determines how any individual will be able to deal with various kinds of problem situations. This global concept has been extremely popular because it has been so successful in a practical sense. Most of our best tests still give us single estimates of intelligence. However, this sort of assumption leaves no room for postulating that a number of independent capacities make up the mental organization and that the same individual may have a high capacity for one type of function but a poor capacity for another. We shall see that this is exactly what has been proposed by some present-day theorists. In the following sections we shall discuss the main theoretical points of view which have been held concerning the nature of intelligence.

Faculty Psychology: We have stated in the historical introduction that, in the eighteenth and nineteenth centuries, considerable interest was awakening in the problems of mental deficiency. The philosophers had already written and speculated a great deal concerning the nature of the intellect. The elemental unit of the mental organization was thought of as sensations which by combination and association were organized into perceptions. These perceptions could be still further elaborated and generalized into concepts. The function of the intellect was considered to be the building of perceptions out of sensations and the construction of conceptions from perceptions.

To accomplish its abstract function, the mind had at its disposal a number of "faculties" such as memory, judgment, attention, reasoning, imagination, etc. These faculties were thought to be like muscles which could be developed by exercise. For example, if a man exercised his faculty of judgment on one problem, the effect of this practice would be to improve his judgment for any other kind of problem. This elaboration of the idea of mental faculties was called the doctrine of "formal discipline," and it influenced education almost up to the present time.

In the early twentieth century Thorndike and Woodworth did the most to eliminate the doctrine of formal discipline from sophisticated thinking by their experiments on transfer of training. But the conceptions of faculty psychology remained a strong influence on theoretical thinking. This influence was one of the reasons that the sensory-motor tests resisted for a long time the European preference for measuring more complex functions in predicting intelligence. The sensory-motor test appeared to many psychologists as the atom (or basic unit) of the mental faculty through which the process of organization of sensations and perceptions could be studied. The theory of faculties was quite incompatible with the concept of general intelligence which was to follow.

The Two-factor Theory: In 1904 Spearman published his first analysis of intelligence. This work was essentially statistical in nature and was further elaborated and revised in the abilities of man. Spearman believed that all intellectual activity contained some element or factor in common. This G, or general factor, was postulated to be important in every mental act, although some acts were thought to depend upon it more than others. The difference between people in intelligence was a matter of how much G they possessed. This general factor Spearman called "mental energy." The variation in measured intelligence that was not explainable in terms of this general factor was attributed by Spearman to specific factors, or S. There were many different specific factors. Those which occurred in a large number of different acts of a particular type, but not all of them, were called group factors. Not only did individuals differ in the strength of the G factor, and therefore in their amount of intelligence, but they also had different kinds and amounts of S factors. Because of this, there were great individual differences in the patterns of ability. Two people of the same general intellectual level might be found to have very different talents and deficiencies. But the important thing for Spearman was how much of this general factor they had.

Spearman's analysis of intelligence was actually an interpretation of certain observations which anyone can make. The theory grew out of the observation that there are correlations between the various measurements of intellectual performance. If a large series of different kinds of intelligence test items like memory, reasoning, perceiving relationships, etc., were given to many people, all the intercorrelations for this series of tests could be arranged in what is called a "correlation matrix.". Using a statistical method of his own invention, the tetrad-difference method, Spearman claimed that he could account for the largest part of the intercorrelations among the tests by one common factor.

Table 4.1. Intercorrelations of Subtests

Subtests	1	2	3	4	5	6	7
1. Analogies	...	.50	.49	.55	.49	.45	.45
2. Completion	.50	...	.54	.47	.50	.38	.34
3. Understanding paragraphs	.49	.54	...	.49	.39	.44	.35
4. Opposites	.55	.47	.49	...	.41	.32	.35
5. Instructions	.49	.28	.39	.41	...	.32	.40
6. Resemblances	.45	.38	.44	.32	.32	...	.35
7. Inferences	.48	.34	.35	.35	.40	.35	

His early work with the tetrad-difference technique for testing the independence of correlations led to the formulation of the two-factor theory of intelligence.

The Multifactor Theory: One of the sharpest critics of Spearman's two factor theory was E. L. Thorndike. Thorndike believed that the intercorrelations studied by Spearman were often too small to test the question of a common factor. Moreover, he disagreed with Spearman in his interpretation of the existing observations. He objected very strongly to the idea of the existence of a characteristic such as general intelligence. Instead of one kind of factor, he maintained that there are a large number of separate characteristics which make up intelligence. He argued that there is no generality to intelligence, but rather communality in the acts that people perform. The common element does not reside in the individual but in the nature of the tasks themselves. People differ in their ability to perform any specific act, that is, in terms of the level of difficulty they can manage. They also differ in the range or number of tasks they can perform. For Thorndike, intelligence was more like a series of skills or talents. Several or many tasks may call for the same kind of ability. The correlations between various tests are the result of the fact that the tests have features in common with each other even though they are called measures of different things.

At first glance Thorndike 's theory appears to be a thoroughly atomistic one. Intelligence is said to be composed of a large number of separate factors or elements. There is no general intelligence but very specific acts. The number of these depends upon how broad or narrow a classification one can or wants to make. However, some tasks have so many elements in common that it is desirable to classify them into groups. We could classify tasks into such categories as arithmetical reasoning, visual perception, word meaning, etc. Despite the atomistic theoretical approach, Thorndike has actually seen fit to classify intellectual activity into three broad types: social intelligence, concrete intelligence, and abstract intelligence. Notice that this is a classification of types of tasks and not an analysis of the mental organization itself. For Thorndike the mental organization consists of a multitude of simple intellectual acts.

We shall see later that this discrepancy of point of view between Spearman and Thorndike is basically a theoretical one and does not greatly affect what one does in the actual measurement of intelligence. The types of tasks which interested Thorndike are essentially the same as the measures which Spearman threw into his correlation matrix.

We might note that among the other critics of Spearman is G. H. Thompson, who has argued that the intercorrelations between tests are the result of common samplings of independent factors. If the tests incorporate many of these independent factors in common (i.e., the tests are all measuring some of the same factors), they will be highly intercorrelated and it will appear as though they are measuring one general factor. This concept is similar to Thorndike's, but unlike Thorndike, Thompson accepted the practical value of the concept of G.

The Factorial Approach: In about 1927, L. L. Thurstone undertook an approach to the study of intelligence which was based upon the analysis of intercorrelations between the various tests of intelligence along the lines of Spearman's earlier work. Using improved techniques of statistical analysis, Thurstone came to vastly different conclusions from Spearman about the nature of intelligence. He published an intelligence test based on the results of his factor analysis and has continued to work along these lines up to the present time. Recently Raymond Cattell has extended the factor analysis techniques to the study of personality. It is unnecessary to attempt an exposition of the factorial techniques here. This is a subject which is discussed at length by most major textbooks on testing and statistics. In short, the technique seeks to determine and define the minimum number of variables or factors which will account for all or most of the variation in intellectual performance.

The procedure, as in the case of Spearman's analysis, involves the presentation of large batteries of intelligence tests to large numbers of subjects. Ideally these tests should comprise all the possible types of measurements that psychologists could agree are related to intelligence. Tests which correlate highly with other tests are measuring some of the same things, while tests which have little or no relationship have nothing in common. Consequently, by the appropriate statistical analysis of the correlation matrix, it is possible to extract a number of factors or variables which have nothing in common with each other but which together account for most of the variation in intellectual performance. By inspection of the tests which have the largest amount of any particular factor (high inter correlations), the factor analyst then attempts to give that variable a name which best describes the function measured.

The series of factors which are extracted from a correlation matrix do not all have the same importance. Some of them account for more of the variation in performance than others. The first factor which is extracted is the one which accounts for the greatest proportion of the total variability. The remaining variation is called the first residual from which a second factor is extracted, then a third, and so on until most or all of the variability is accounted for or until the residuals are not large enough to make further extraction of factors worth while.

In his writings on the subject Thurstone argued that intellectual performance was an expression of a number of factors rather than a common general factor. For him the goal of intelligence test construction should be the isolation of the primary factors and the construction of tests which measure individually each of these factors. In his earlier work Thurstone announced a number of factors which he believed made up intellectual performance. These were identified as spatial (S), perceptual (P), numerical (N), verbal relations (V), memory (M), word fluency (W), induction (I), reasoning (R), and deduction (D). In later studies there has been some modification of this list. In 1943, for example, Thurstone listed six factors, with induction eliminated altogether, and perceptual and deductive uncertain.

Summary and Overview

For convenience in thinking it is possible to place the three theoretical approaches to the nature of the mental organization on a continuum. At one extreme lies the atomistic view of Thorndike which stresses a large number of mental elements. These separate elements act in combination in any mental act and may seem to be general in nature because of common elements among the various intellectual tasks that people are required to do. At the other extreme is the global concept of Spearman which suggests that some general quality of the mental organization pervades every mental act even though there may be specific abilities which determine the unique quality of a particular individual's performance. And finally, between these two falls Thurstone 's views that not one general factor, nor a large number of specific factors, but a small number of independent factors make up the mental process.

All three points of view begin with somewhat different assumptions about the mental organization. Consequently they reason differently about the essentially similar data which they are analyzing. From the same correlational matrix it is possible to arrive at these opposing beliefs since the data themselves do not directly answer the question. Even the tests which Thurstone designed to be measures of the independent factors of intelligence are correlated with one another, which suggests that some additional factor or factors are contained in the measures. In an effort to be eclectic it has been proposed by some that Spearman's G corresponds to Thurstone 's first primary factor. In any case the question of the adequacy of the three theories to explain all the facts remains unsettled.

In discussing the factorial approach to intelligence it might be well to refer to some studies on the relationship of age to the intercorrelation between intellectual factors such as verbal, numerical, and spatial. Garrett presented controversial evidence that in children there appears to be more evidence of a general factor (higher inter correlations) such as Spearman suggested, than in adulthood. Garrett writes, "The conclusion which I draw from these data is that the over-all ability (g) which looms large during the elementary school years becomes progressively less important at the high school and college level, where factor studies have shown it to be negligible or quite small." At the high-school and college levels, abstract intelligence appears to become dismembered into specific components or more independent factors. Later research and critical reviews of Garrett's concept essentially discredit this point of view. Failure to control such factors as task difficulty and differing variability at different age levels probably account for Garrett's finding. The dismemberment concept can probably not be adequately tested for methodological reasons, although it is an interesting attempt to bring together the Spearman and Thurstone points of view.

One of the chief limitations in the approaches discussed above concerns the fact that the correlation matrix from which all three theories are derived depends upon what tests are included.

Intelligence is what we call certain kinds of activities which we can measure only through certain kinds and samples of behavior. The tasks one includes to measure these behaviors depend upon many complex considerations, not the least of which is one's cultural frame of reference. The entire argument may tend to become circular, since the types of tests we include depend on our prior notion of what intelligence is. For example, if the correlation matrix contains no tests which depend on speed, then speed will not appear as a factor in our factor analysis. However, if we have decided in advance that speed is one of the variables our tests should measure, then it may appear as an important source of variation in our battery of tests.

The factor analysts do not claim that the number of factors is fixed or even known. This point has not always been made clear. There is no doubt that the adequacy of this type of analysis depends entirely upon the appropriateness of the measures one selects in the first place. We are always dealing with a limited sample of behavior. This fact has been the primary criticism of factor analysis. The objections do not tend to lie with the statistics but with the raw data themselves. This argument applies to all three of the theoretical approaches. Examination of the intercorrelations will not put into the formula what is not already there. It has been suggested that these limitations reduce all three of the approaches to mere conceptual models on which to pattern our thinking and that the real nature of intelligence cannot be understood by factorial methods. Few people deny, however, that such models are useful, or even at times necessary, for research into the problem of the nature of intelligence.

One way in which to judge the importance of the differences between the theoretical views concerning the nature of intelligence is to study how these points of view affect the construction of tests. Let us look at the kinds of tests advocated by the proponents of each theory.

While Thorndike sees intelligence as made up of a multitude of minute elements of ability, he recognizes that this concept is not so significant in a practical sense as the idea that many of these elements operate together in a task which requires intelligent behavior. Some of these elements may be grouped in one class because they are found in one broad kind of intellectual activity. For example, one of Thorndike's best known tests was designed to measure the ability of people to handle abstract concepts, one broad category of mental effort. The CAVD Test consists of four parts: the sentence completion (C), arithmetical reasoning (A), vocabulary (V), and following directions (D). According to Thorndike this test does not measure all the elements in abstract intelligence. The other aspects of abstract intelligence not measured directly can be estimated because of the high correlations between performance on all abstract tasks. As we shall see, this test contains the same kinds of items that may be found in the great majority of current tests which provide some single measure of over-all intelligence. These current tests, as does the CAVD, tend to give a heavy weighting to what is called abstract intelligence. Thorndike's views in practice do not, therefore, lead to radically different types of tests than we are accustomed to use.

Since Spearman argues for a general factor of intelligence and includes in his correlation matrix the same kinds of tests that are used today in the clinic to measure intelligence, no alteration of our popular system of providing a single estimate of intellectual capacity is called for by his theoretical approach. The best test, says Spearman, is one which calls for the largest amount of the general factor, and the best test materials should therefore be those which have high intercorrelations. Each part of the test should be so thoroughly saturated with the general factor that the effects of the specific factors would be canceled out. This recommendation of Spearman tends to be the actual practice today (viz., the Stanford-Binet, whose subtests are highly intercorrelated), although many psychologists are recommending that a single estimate of intelligence be abandoned.

The extreme practical conclusion that one would draw from the assumptions of Thurstone concerning the nature of intelligence is at great odds with the implications of either Thorndike 's or Spearman's theories. For the factor analyst, any single measure of intellectual capacity is inappropriate. What we should be obtaining is a profile showing the individual's performance in the various primary factors which have been established by factorial technique. Psychologists with this point of view argue that we are not justified in adding up test items correctly passed in these various functions and that a total score representing intelligence is not meaningful.

In following this orientation, Thurstone has introduced his Primary Mental Abilities Tests. Even these tests embody content which is basically similar to the tests which have been constructed out of the other theoretical frames of reference. They tend to contain material which measures academic and abstract abilities. They have not proved to be especially useful to the clinician as yet, and their future in a practical sense is difficult to predict. The importance of this approach may increase with greater interest in the effects of pathology on the various kinds of intellectual functioning.

Let us now summarize the discussion of the relationship between theory and practice. We have first noted that, while differing greatly in theory, Thorndike's and Spearman's concepts led to similar types of tests with the tendency to use a single measure to express intellectual level. On the other hand, Thurstone's approach rejected the single measure of intelligence in favor of a profile, although he used the same types of tasks as were employed by Thorndike and Spearman. At the present time, what one does in the clinic with regard to the measurement of intelligence does not depend greatly upon theoretical position. Although a number of psychologists have predicted changes in the near future, nearly all our standard tests give single measures of intellectual level. The practical value of pure factor tests (which are virtually impossible to achieve) may be in the future. The main impact of Thurstone's approach has been at the theoretical level.

In the early days of modern psychology the opinion was held that mental acts should be divided into three types: cognitive, conative, and affective. The cognitive aspect referred to the process of knowing and included only the intellectual functions. The conative side of mental acts included all aspects of motivation. The term "affective" was used to designate the emotional side of behavior. Psychology developed the tendency to study these components of behavior independently of each other, or at least, with the tendency to think of them separately. While some psychologists today are arguing that this is no longer a justifiable way to approach psychological problems, present-day thinking is still greatly influenced by this division. Although no one would ever have argued that problem-solving behavior did not require motivation, it is interesting that all our measurements attempt to isolate intelligence from its motivational component. In effect, we have been trying to study intelligence with motivation and emotions controlled.

At an early stage, in attempting to understand a very complex process, this over simple kind of classification is often convenient. The principal objection to this way of proceeding in the study of human intelligence is that it may actually lead us to overlook the nature of the total mental act. We are gradually moving away from the extreme position that there are such things as cognitive functions which are separate and distinct from affective and motivational ones. Those psychologists who are still willing to separate cognitive from affective and conative are beginning to speak of interactions between them. Others go even further and suggest that the distinction should be dropped altogether in our thinking.

Recognition of these considerations has led a number of psychologists to talk about what have been called "non intellective factors" in intelligence. Wechsler, in a presidential address to the Division of Clinical and Abnormal Psychology, discussed some of the thinking along these lines. He pointed out that, when the correlation matrices of intelligence tests are factored, only about 60 per cent of the total variability in the test performance is ever accounted for by the factors. Moreover, factor analysts, some of them from Spearman's own laboratory, have been able to demonstrate the existence of factors which seem to be nonintellectual in nature. Interpreting evidence from a number of kinds of sources, Wechsler concludes that " general intelligence is the function of the personality as a whole and is determined by emotion and conative factors."

Writers other than Wechsler have also made this point. Goodenough has stated the problem clearly in a brief exposition of what she has called "the mathematical analysis of nonintellectual traits." She writes,

> *That such factors as self-control, level of aspiration, interest and zest in achievement, and a host of other matters by which potential abilities are either energized or constricted in their manifestations play an important part both in performance on mental tests and in the larger problems of real life is generally admitted. As yet, however, work in this area has not advanced far beyond the level of single measurements; little has been done to show the organization of these non-intellectual traits either with respect to each other or -- what may perhaps be more important -- with respect to their integration with the abilities and achievements of*

the individual. Common observation indicates that a basic problem in the field of human behavior is involved in such relationships. How often do we hear such pronouncements as these: "He could if he would, but he won't make the effort." "He's not very clever, to be sure, but he never gives up till he gets there." "He is a good workman but he can't hold a job because of his bad temper." Regardless of the accuracy of the particular statements, the general principle is beyond question.

Before leaving the theoretical issues surrounding the problem of the nature of intelligence, something should be said about the classical nature-nurture question. Many different points of view have been held concerning the relative influence of hereditary and environmental factors in intellectual behavior. The question has prompted a fair amount of research, usually by the co-twin method of studying the influence of environment. In this method heredity is controlled through the use of identical twins. None of these studies has ever really settled the issue. In view of what we have said about the inappropriateness of separating the cognitive, conative, and affective side of mental performance, the question really has very little meaning. We do not strictly measure capacity with our intelligence tests. We are measuring a person's performance which is the end product of many variables. We have pointed out that motivation, personality characteristics like persistence and self-confidence, chemical factors related to metabolism, and other variables enter into the measurement of the individual's intelligence. Unless these variables are isolated in our measurement, we cannot hope to assess the role of genes or biological factors in intellectual performance. The evidence is such that one can take almost any point of view concerning the nature nurture question.

Because of the above considerations and other questions which we have not treated here, a great many psychologists have preferred to soft-pedal the issue of heredity and environment in intelligence. We tend to say that both hereditary and environmental variables, whose operation we do not fully understand, interact in any individual's intellectual performance. In some instances environmental circumstances may appear more important, while in others hereditary factors stand out. However, making this sort of statement, or labeling any case of mental retardation or acceleration as hereditary or environmental in nature, does not solve the problem of understanding the nature of intellectual performance. In general, the nature-nurture question has not been productive in bringing us closer to an understanding of human intelligence.

In some of the introductory texts on psychology, or in other introductory sources, the student is likely to come across a topic which is usually called the "constancy of the IQ." It has been pointed out that an individual's intelligence quotient remains stable throughout life, that is, his brightness or rate of mental growth does not change. A child who has an IQ of 120 at 10 years of age will have roughly the same IQ at 13. A great deal has been made of this point, and the impression is often gained that the IQ represents a person's inherent ability which is uninfluenced by any environmental conditions. In passing we would like to comment on this notion of the IQ's constancy.

In the first place, it should be clear by now that the IQ or any other measure of intelligence is not a measure of an individual's inherent capacity. It is considerably influenced by education and, as we have labored long to point out, by the personality of the individual. Moreover, the IQ at different ages does not have exactly the same meaning. For statistical reasons related to problems of measurement, it is more difficult to obtain an IQ of 120 at 13 or 14 years of age than it is to achieve such a score at 9 or 10.

Because of the misunderstandings wrought by the various claims about the constancy of the IQ, we believe it is necessary to point out just what is really meant by such a statement. If the IQ as a measure of mental alertness or brightness is to be useful to us, it must, of course, be reasonably stable. This is actually the case. Within reasonable limits the IQ does not vary greatly. But it does vary some, and ignorance of this fact has led people into making foolish statements. Its relative constancy, even taking account of environmental factors and the deficits of old age, is one of its chief virtues since it does make possible the consistent measurement of mental alertness throughout a good part of the life of the person. The measurement of intelligence has been one of the most useful enterprises of psychologists. From time to time researchers have claimed that chemical treatment of the feebleminded produced a change in the IQ. Others have argued that it was possible to train a person's intelligence so that the IQ would be raised. Positive findings in some of these studies have sometimes led to the belief that the question of heredity or environment had been solved, since it was possible to change a person's intellectual level by certain physical or psychological methods.

There is no question that IQ variations will occur. These variations are a function of the nature of the measuring devices which we use to estimate ability. Some change will occur, for example, if you train children on the kinds of intellectual tasks that are found on tests like the Stanford-Binet. This does not mean, however, that we have altered the individual's basic intelligence. Moreover, psychotherapy or psychological support with children who are anxious or disturbed will often produce IQ changes which mean simply that such children have been made more effective in their performance because of the removal of crippling emotional difficulties. The attention given to such children may well act to change their confidence level or motivation to succeed at the tasks found on the tests.

Indeed, because the measurement of intellectual performance is so reliable, it becomes possible to assess the contribution of factors such as education, social conditions, senescence, etc., to intellectual performance. The vulnerability of these intelligence measures to the effects of personality and social variables need not be looked upon as a liability. Intelligence measurement offers a means of studying the relationship of cognitive performance to emotional and motivational conditions.

Aside from the theoretical interest in the nature of intellectual behavior, the clinician is concerned with what his tests will do in a practical way. He is faced with certain questions about the patient, and he must find instruments which allow him to make accurate predictions. Making predictions from tests demands that the test correlate with the behavior to be predicted to an extent which makes such a prediction practical. The expert clinical psychologist will not usually make such a prediction on the basis of a single test but tries to diagnose on the basis of as much relevant information as he has available. As a consequence, he often makes a mental adjustment in his diagnoses, which accounts for the factors that our intelligence tests do not adequately measure. He may say, "This man has the ability but lacks the maturity and persistence to be a good graduate student." But the essential assumption behind his use of tests of intelligence is that they correlate to some extent with the criterion measure or behavior which he desires to predict.

Most of our usable tests give some single index of general intelligence. They follow the Binet orientation of being validated against academic grades. Typically, the best tests of intelligence correlate with school grades to the extent of about .50 or .60. In selected populations with a restricted range of talent, as in graduate school, these relationships may be much smaller. This means that in individual prediction considerable error will be made. Nevertheless it is possible to make better guesses by using these tests than could be made without them. Moreover, this correlation may be raised by the inclusion of other kinds of information about the individual. Measures of intelligence, however limited, are of great help when we are trying to understand the reasons for a person's failure in school or when we are concerned with the problem of school placement. There is no doubt, however, that many clinicians misuse these tests. It is important to understand at least the practical limitations of a test score before that score can be properly interpreted.

We shall see a little later that even our tests of general intelligence may give us much more information than a single score. They may allow us to discover the kinds of functions in which an individual is especially advanced or deficient. They may also allow us to examine the qualitative features of a person's performance from which we can make guesses about the nonintellective factors such as persistence, self-confidence, flexibility of approach, and so on. These guesses may increase our practical ability to understand the patient's problem or predict his future behavior.

Aptitude and Achievement

There are many times when we are interested in predicting the success of an individual or group of people in learning some specific skill. In order to make this prediction, more information about the person may be needed than an intelligence score. As a matter of fact, intelligence test results might tell us very little about a man's potential skill in a particular sphere like music. Tests which are specifically designed to allow us to predict future proficiency in a particular skill are called "aptitude" tests. Their most frequent uses are in vocational guidance and in personnel selection. Tests of specific aptitudes have been designed to measure potential skill in a very large variety of fields. Mechanical aptitude, clerical aptitude, musical aptitude, and medical-school aptitude are only a small number of examples.

The student of psychological testing is often confused by the distinction between aptitude and intelligence. As he examines the various tests, he may find striking similarities between some aptitude tests and intelligence tests. He discovers that the American Council on Education Psychological Test is called a college aptitude test because the skill to be predicted is success in college. "But," he asks, "aren't intelligence tests usually validated against school grades? What, then, is the actual difference between tests of aptitude and tests of intelligence?" In a practical sense there is often great overlap between tests of intelligence and some aptitude tests. This is particularly true in the case of aptitude tests which specifically attempt to predict academic success as in the case of the ACE. In other cases the overlap is very slight, as with tests of clerical aptitude. The distinctions between aptitude and intelligence are not clear-cut.

Some writers have abandoned the use of the term "aptitude" because of this ambiguity. The main difference between the two classes of measures may be summarized in two points. In the first place, aptitude tests tend to be narrow in scope, that is, limited to performance on a particular skill. For example, the Seashore Tests of Musical Talent attempt to measure discrimination of pitch, loudness, time, timbre, rhythm, and memory for tones, which are thought by the author to be fundamental capacities for success in a musical occupation. These talents could hardly be predicted by a test of intelligence, although they may not be entirely independent of it.

The second major difference between aptitude tests and tests of intelligence arises from their dependence upon prior training or experience. The intelligence test is usually constructed so that people will have a reasonably equal chance of performing well regardless of such factors as schooling or past experience. While intelligence tests do not altogether succeed at this effort, they are, by and large, freer from this confounding than are the aptitude tests. In aptitude measurement psychologists are always primarily concerned with producing a practical instrument which will give them the maximal predicting power regardless of the theoretical basis of that prediction.

As we have found with aptitude and intelligence, there is also great overlap between intelligence and tests of achievement. The achievement test is aimed at measuring what a person has already learned in some special area, rather than predicting future progress. When a student takes a final examination in a course in school, he is taking an achievement test. One of its purposes is to tell the instructor how much a student has absorbed of the course work so that he can give him a grade. In the same way a standardized achievement test is given to determine how much mathematics, literature, reading skill, and so on, a person may have learned. In this way it is possible to find out the strong and weak points in a person's training and possibly apply corrective measures if they are called for.

Tests of Intelligence

In this section we shall list samples of the various kinds of intelligence tests and briefly discuss some of them. The list will not be a complete one by any means, since it would be impossible and undesirable to give a full description in this book of all the tests of intelligence which are available. However, we have made an effort to include representative tests in each area and particularly those which are of the greatest use to the clinician.

Intelligence Tests at Different Chronological Ages

Infant Tests . Psychologists have attempted to extend the techniques of intelligence testing to infants. The age range included here generally goes up to 18 months or 2 years. This is the period when speech has not developed to a sufficient degree to allow much social intercourse. The earliest important contribution to this field was made by Gesell, who introduced the first set of infant tests of development as a result of the elaborate observation of large numbers of infants of all ages.

In the main, tests for this age range have not proved very successful as predictors of later intellectual development. Infants are difficult to test. Verbal instructions make little sense to the child. Their motivation is uncertain, and their attention is difficult to

Table 4.1. The Constancy of Mental Test Performance in the Guidance and Control Group

Age			Stanford-Binet							
			2-0	2-6	3-0	3-6	4-0	5-0	6-0	7-0
	Group	N	r	r	R	r	r	r	r	r
1-9	Guidance	117	.68±.04	.59±.04	.47±.05	.50±.05	.46±.05	.32±.06	.30±.06	.42±.06
	Control	117			.59±.04	.47±.05	.33±.06	.43±.06	.30±.06	.19±.07
2-0	Guidance	113		.71±.03	.69±.03	.60±.04	.46±.05	.32±.06	.47±.05	.46±.05
2-6	Guidance	114			.73±.03	.64±.04	.57±.05	.46±.05	.37±.06	.38±.06
3-0	Guidance	116				.73±.03	.64±.04	.53±.05	.54±.05	.56±.05
	Control	113				.71±.03	.59±.04	.60±.04	.60±.04	.54±.05
3-6	Guidance	107					.78±.03	.72±.03	.59±.04	.63±.04
	Control	108					.74±.03	.71±.03	.62±.04	.59±.04
4-0	Guidance	105						.69±.04	.61±.04	.66±.04
	Control	106						.75±.03	.62±.04	.53±.05
5-0	Guidance	104							.65±.04	.73±.03
	Control	106							.77±.03	.72±.03
S.B.	Guidance	109								.81±.02
6-0	Control	105								.83±.02
S.B.	Guidance	104								
7-0	Control	104								

control. There is the question of whether there is such a thing as measurable intelligence before speech has appeared. The accuracy of such measures is also questionable because of the rapid rate of development in all spheres which makes each small age difference count for so much. Correlations between the Stanford-Binet given at 3 years or older and infant tests given between the ages of 12 to 18 months have been noted by Goodenough to range from .35 to .65. In most instances they are too low to avoid large errors in individual prediction.

The types of performance found in the tests of infant development include such functions as coordination, simple vocalization, attention to test objects, simple block building, manipulation, and so forth. Some of the better known infant tests are: Bayley's California First Year Mental Scale, Cattell's Intelligence Scale for Infants and Young Children which is an extension of the Stanford-Binet to the infant level, and the Buhler Baby-Tests.

Preschool Tests: The age range for these tests runs from about 18 months to about 5 years. Shyness, negativism, lack of interest, and lack of comprehension of the purpose of the tests are serious handicaps in obtaining valid measures at this time of life. The kinds of items found in these tests, depending upon the age and ability of the child, include more complex block building, language comprehension, pegboards, information, picture puzzles, vocabulary, and digit spans.

The correlations between the preschool tests and later estimates of intelligence using the Stanford-Binet increase steadily with advancing age when the preschool test was given. Honzik has presented a table which shows this relationship.

These data mean that, for the preschool age range, the older the child is when tested, the closer to later intelligence scores will be the estimate of intelligence derived.

The following are some of the best known tests of intelligence for preschool children: the Stanford-Binet contains items which extend as low as 2 years; the Cattell Intelligence Scale for Infants and Young Children goes up to 41/2 years; the Merrill-Palmer Scale and the Minnesota Pre-school Scales are other examples.

The full list is actually a large one. Hildreth lists 33 such tests at the preschool level. The tests which have been mentioned above are all administered individually. It is not feasible to test young children in groups until they have had at least some school or kindergarten experience. Under some conditions it is possible to use tests like the Goodenough Draw a Man Test in small groups. The Thurstones have also devised an intelligence test for children, based on their factorial techniques, which may be given in groups. This test is called the Thurstone Primary Abilities Tests for Ages Five and Six. It has not achieved wide popularity.

School-age Tests: During this period of life (approximately 7 to 15 years of age), children are usually easier to test than at any other time. They have gained a strong sense of competition and are generally cooperative. They are not likely to become suspicious of the purpose of the testing and are less self-conscious about their performance. Test results are likely to be more valid during this period because of these considerations as well as because the appropriate tests have been more carefully standardized and experimented upon than those available for other age ranges. Moreover, the performance of the testees is less likely to come so close to the highest or lowest levels possible that the resulting measurement will be unreliable.

For persons of school age and older, it is possible to separate verbal and nonverbal abilities and to use group as well as individual tests. The types of tests at this period of life merge with the types found in the measurement of adult capacity. In the sections which follow we shall discuss individual, group, verbal, and performance types of tests.

Individual Tests

Verbal: For many years after the publication by Goddard of the simple Binet test there have been a number of revisions of this instrument. Binet himself published one in 1908 which was later translated by Goddard. Goddard revised this latter test in 1911.

In his last revision Kuhlmann recommended the use of an altogether different index of intelligence than the IQ. For the concept of mental age Kuhlmann substituted mental units. This quantity was based upon a curve of mental growth developed by Heinis. Both Heinis and Kuhlmann believed that this curve represented the true course of mental development. The mental units (MU) score could be converted into an index called the per cent of average (PA) which was in some ways like the IQ. However, the PA represented the MU score (that is, the average level of difficulty of the problems which the child could pass) divided by the average MU score for that individual's own age level (obtained by testing large numbers of children of the same age). Like the IQ, indexes which exceeded unity indicated a greater than average mental development. A PA below 1 meant that the child did not have the mental development which was expected (average) for his chronological age. In contrast to the PA, the IQ requires dividing the mental age score by the chronological age of the individual. The principle of an index of brightness is basic to the two techniques, and consequently, despite their differences statistically, both the PA and IQ are interpreted similarly.

Kuhlmann 's test also differed from the original Binet test in that it was a point scale rather than an age scale. In the Binet test the subtests are grouped by age levels. Heterogeneous items (like reasoning, vocabulary, memory, etc.) are grouped together in the same age level because they are of similar difficulty. In the point scale a homogeneous collection of items are grouped together (reasoning alone, etc.). These items are arranged in order of increasing difficulty. The child completes one kind of item as far as he can go up the scale of difficulty, and then he goes on to another kind of item, say memory, beginning again with easy items. Each item has an age value and, in the Kuhlmann revision, a value in mental units. This enables the examiner to determine the mental level of the individual by averaging the number of mental units obtained by the child throughout the scale.

Among psychologists interested in the problems of intelligence testing, there has been a great deal of discussion about the relative merits of the age scale as compared with the point scale. The point scale has generally been preferred. The same kind of controversy has occurred over Kuhlmann 's PA as opposed to the Binet use of the IQ. Whatever the merits of either technique, the Kuhlmann scale is rarely used today, and Kuhlmann 's terms, MU and PA, are seldom referred to except in a historical sense.

Concerning the use of such measures as the IQ and the PA, neither of these statistics is really the most accurate way of portraying an individual's intellectual brightness. The standard score, based upon normal-curve statistics, is considered to be the most appropriate way to describe an individual's standing in any group. Most testers agree, however, that the concept of the IQ has stuck in our usage because of its wide dissemination among educators and the public. For children under the age of 15 the IQ is reasonably adequate, and any attempt to substitute ordinary standard scores would no doubt be met with considerable opposition. As unfortunate as this is, it appears that we will have to go along with the old-fashioned IQ for some time to come.

In addition to Goddard's and Kuhlmann 's work, the Binet scale was revised by Yerkes and others in 1915 and 1923 as a point scale with its own innovations. In 1922 Herring introduced another point-scale revision. Terman, in 1916, at Stanford University, constructed the Stanford Revision of the Binet-Simon Intelligence Scale, which rapidly became popular, and then in 1937, with Merrill, he published a larger, more useful, and better standardized version. The original Stanford revision and the more recent 1937 replacement have never had any real competition among individual verbal intelligence tests for elementary school children. Although it is an age scale, for the clinician working with children it is the verbal intelligence test. Because of its importance to clinical work with children, it has sometimes been overemphasized in terms of the time spent with it in the training of the present-day clinical psychologist.

The Stanford-Binet scale consists of a large number of items which range from 2 years to the superior adult level. The younger children are given such tasks as stringing wooden beads, naming common objects, block building, etc. Throughout the test at the later levels are found such items as memory for words, numbers, and paragraphs; vocabulary; finding absurdities; identifying similarities; and other tasks involving information, perception, reasoning, memory, and verbal facility. The test has two forms, Form L and Form M, which are different in content but are relatively equivalent in other essential respects so that a child may be retested at some later date.

For a complete description and evaluation of the Stanford-Binet the reader should refer to any acceptable textbook on testing. Excellent accounts may be found in Cronbach and Freeman. For the original material and a detailed description of the tests, the scoring system, and the standardization, Terman and Merrill should be consulted.

While there is no need to duplicate this material here, some main points of evaluation should be made concerning the test. This is based in part on the fact that considerable care went into its standardization and construction. The test offers great variety in the battery of subtests. A wealth of observational data of the manner in which the child attacks intellectual problems may be obtained during the testing. It is an interesting test for children. Of some special value is the fact that clinicians, educators, and the lay public at large are more familiar with this test than any other instrument, and an enormous body of experience with and information about the test has been accumulated over the many years of its popularity. Even a superior test to the 1937 revision would have a difficult time competing with it. A halo seems to surround it. It has even been used as a criterion against which to estimate the validity of new tests of intelligence. However, the limitations of the test are great, and it is probable that with our gradually changing concepts of intellectual capacity newer instruments of a different type will emerge.

It is of paramount importance to understand what the Stanford-Binet actually measures. We shall mention here the main questions concerning the interpretation of the tests results.

1. The Binet test does not measure innate ability. No test does. It is heavily loaded with verbal items and is certainly influenced greatly by educational and cultural experiences. The standardization of the test was based upon children in the American culture, largely urban. This means that the test has limited or no usefulness with other cultural groups. Despite this, people have spent many hours in vain attempting to determine intellectual differences between various national and racial groups. Even its use with bilinguals, Negroes, and whites from impoverished social areas is dangerous.
2. When the intelligence score is interpreted, many examiners fail to recognize that it is highly influenced by non intellective factors. Confounded together in his performance is the child's persistence, flexibility, self-confidence, inhibitions, and other personality variables. It is a great mistake to assume that we have measured pure intellectual capacity when personality characteristics partly determine performance. The skilled

clinician is always on the alert for qualitative features in the examination record which give him clues about these personality variables. These clues allow him to more fully appraise the test.

Comprehension items
Age 3 year 6 months
What must you do when you are thirty
Why do we have storms
Age 4 year
Why do we have booms?
Age 2 year
What's the thing for you to do when you have broken something which belongs to someone else?

Psychomotor items
Age 3 year
Child must using at least four heads
Child must copy satisfactorily a circle with pencil and paper.
Age 5 year
Child must copy satisfactorily a square with pencil and paper.
Age 6 year
Child must copy a simple pattern in making a beads chain of at least four beads e.g.
Age 9 year
Child must draw two figures from memory

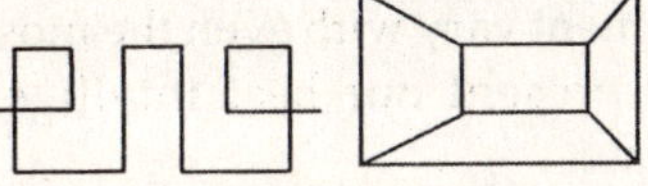

Miscalls item
Age 4 year 6 months
Child must repeat one list of 4 digits correctly: a) 4-7-2-9-; b) 3-8-5-2; c) 7-2-6-1.
Age 7 year Child must correctly identify the similarity between at least two of the pairs of object. In what way these thinks alike?

Fig. 4.1. Examples of Items on the Stanford-Binet.

3. There are important disadvantages in a test which provides a single index of mental ability and which does not provide us with separate measures of different kinds of intellectual functioning. The Binet-type tests contain a mixture of many elements, most of which are substantially inter correlated. It is difficult to attempt to identify, within the same subject, the

adequacy of intellectual functioning in various areas like reasoning, memory, information, etc. Clinical testing is shifting gradually into the practice of attempting to separate out the various mental functions. There is an increasing tendency to ask, "In what areas is the individual deficient and in which does he excel?" Many psychologists would agree that there are different kinds of intelligence not all of which are measured by any test. This kind of approach must depend upon correlational analysis to determine the measures which are reasonably independent of each other.

4. Although the Stanford-Binet has been and is being given on occasion to adults, or late adolescents, it is completely inappropriate for people over 14 or 15 years of age. The standardization population was primarily children, and the IQ is a measure that has no meaning for an adult population.
5. The empirical validity of the Stanford-Binet is not spectacular. Bond lists some correlations found between the test and tenth-grade achievement which are fairly typical of what others have found. With reading comprehension, the correlation is .73; with English and history, .59; with biology,.54; with geometry, .48; and with reading speed, .43. Predictions of academic achievement vary with even the most widely used and probably at present our best intelligence tests are extremely inaccurate.
6. A number of other questions have been raised which apply to measurement problems in intelligence testing in general. The Stanford-Binet is an age scale. As we have already noted, many writers have argued that this type of scale is less adequate than the point scale. Moreover, the IQ has been attacked long and frequently as being a poor measure. Its meaning at different age levels varies because not only do the types of tasks at different age levels differ but the standard error of the IQ is also variable. Competent testers, including Terman, agree that the use of standard scores is superior statistically to any other measure of intellectual performance. However, many of them argue that it would confuse large numbers of people who are not familiar with the concept of standard scores but who understand the IQ. The present authors believe that this

is an unfortunate attitude, since it perpetuates a bad concept on the grounds that it is easier for people to understand than the correct one.

These and other considerations seem to be poorly understood among the great majority of Stanford-Binet users and make for serious errors in interpretation. This is probably the case because the test is widely used by unsophisticated teachers and poorly trained clinicians as well as competent individuals. In the hands of a skilled worker the Binet and the Binet-type test can be of great value. Judgments of feeble-mindedness, although not made properly with a test alone, depend upon Binet-style tests. The detection of personality deviations by means of the quality of responses, the pattern, and the approach to the test situation can result from competent Binet testing. Moreover, decisions about foster-home or school-grade placement are included in the practical applications of the modern versions of the Binet. These and other features make the Stanford-Binet invaluable at present to the clinical worker who is concerned with child problems.

Performance: It is often necessary to obtain an estimate of a person's intellectual level when the use of a test which is heavily weighted with verbal materials is impossible or inappropriate because of language handicaps. Performance tests help to remedy this difficulty by making use of items which call for manipulation rather than verbal responses. Some of these tests require verbal instructions and are sometimes distinguished from true non language tests in which the directions are given in pantomime to avoid completely the use of speech.

There has been a tendency on the part of many clinical psychologists to treat scores derived from performance tests as measures of practical or manipulative ability rather than as a measure of one kind of intelligence. This habit makes performance intelligence a kind of stepsister to the "real intelligence" as measured by the Binet. Consequently, a child may be described as subnormal in intelligence but with excellent practical or manipulative ability. Wechsler and others have commented upon the absurdity of this practice. As a matter of fact, Alexander has suggested that "a perfect performance battery would be a better measure of g than a perfect verbal battery." Alexander makes this comment on the basis of data showing the theoretical G loadings for verbal and performance tests to be .60 and .81, respectively. Interestingly enough, correlations between verbal and performance tests are usually rather low though always positive. Correlations between verbal tests and academic grades are higher than between performance tests and academic ability. Despite the confusion over what they measure in relation to verbal tests, the child psychologist must have some mastery of the performance tests, since they are often an important source of supplementary information concerning the child's intellectual capacity.

The first performance scale was developed in 1917 by Pintner and Paterson, who standardized some of the performance tests earlier experimented with by Healy and Fernald. The latter two, many years earlier, had been interested in devising tests for studying the intellectual levels and personality traits of juvenile delinquents. In 1917 Pintner and Paterson published their scale of 15 tests which could be presented without the use of verbal communication and which did not require the use of language on the part of the testee. The scale was designed for children between the ages of 4 and 15 years. Many of the items of this test were the forerunners of similar or identical items in later performance tests. The test items included picture puzzles, many types of form boards, picture completions, a substitution test, and an order of tapping test.

In 1930 Grace Arthur introduced a restandardization of eight tests of the Pintner-Paterson battery and added two new tests. This instrument is the most popular performance test today. The items added were the well-known Porteus Maze Test and the Kohs Block Design Test. Cornell and Coxe published another performance scale for children in 1934 which differed considerably from the first two, particularly in that it contained none of the form boards which were so prominent in the Pintner-Paterson and the Arthur tests. A few other tests of the form-board type occasionally crop up in clinical use. The Ferguson Form Boards have been designed for very young school children and range up to the college-senior level. The Kent-Shakow Form Boards are primarily for adult use although the standardization population ranges from 6 years to adults. The Grove modification of the Kent-Shakow Form Boards made use of male adult penitentiary prisoners for its standardization.

Performance tests tend to emphasize reasoning behavior involving mostly visual perception. They deemphasize competence in the use of verbal and numerical symbols. As we have noted above, they were originally designed as substitutes for verbal tests like the Binet when such measurement was not feasible. Their reliabilities have tended to be somewhat lower than desirable. Moreover, their correlations with verbal tests of the Binet type have generally been low (lower than .50) when age is held constant.

While the two types of tests, verbal and performance, measure some things in common, it is also apparent that they measure important functions which are different from each other. The Pintner-Paterson and the Arthur Point Scale were designed with the idea of different kinds of intelligence in mind. The authors of the Cornell-Coxe believed that a performance test should not be a substitute for, but a supplement to, the verbal-type test. This point of view has been encouraged by the factor analysts who argue that the performance tests are obviously measuring some of the primary factors which are not found in the verbal tests. They should not be considered simply as tests of manual dexterity or mechanical ability.

Although present-day interpretations of performance test scores are somewhat controversial, they are nevertheless essential in the clinical situation for children with language handicaps. They are the only standardized estimates of intelligence possible with the deaf, the non-English-speaking children, the illiterate, and children with speech disabilities. They also offer interesting opportunities to observe the operation of personality characteristics such as persistence, rashness, confidence, and other presently qualitative features of the child's approach to perceptual-motor tasks. Discrepancies between scores on the performance tests and on the verbal tests lead us to examine the reasons for these differences. In the long run it will be necessary to examine the child's functioning in real-life situations and relate it to the various kinds of intellectual capacities which we measure.

The Wechsler-Bellevue: Although the 1937 Stanford-Binet includes tests for the average and superior adult, it is really inappropriate for adult use. The standardization was based primarily upon a children's population. Besides the IQ is an inappropriate statistic for adults. Until 1939 no other individual intelligence tests of any consequence were available for adult testing. In that year the Wechsler-Bellevue appeared and rapidly gained popularity as the best measure of adult intelligence. The test was standardized for ages 10 to 60. It is still the only adequate individual test for adults which is available. In the modern clinic it ranks with the Binet as one of the most important tools of measurement.

The test is given orally and consists of 10 subtests, 5 verbal in nature and 5 performance, with a separate measure of vocabulary. Two forms of the test are available for retesting. The verbal scale consists of the following subtests:, (1) information, (2) comprehension, (3) arithmetical reasoning, (4) memory span for digits, and (5) similarities. The performance items are quite similar to the tasks found in some of the earlier performance tests for children. They are: (1) picture arrangement, (2) picture completion, (3) block design, (4) object assembly, and (5) digit symbol.

The Wechsler-Bellevue is a point scale: Its score is expressed in terms of an IQ which does not mean the same thing as the Stanford-Binet IQ. It is in reality a standard score with a concession in terminology to popular usage. In this respect (that is, in the use of a single score) the Wechsler assumes some general intellectual factor. The intertest correlations are relatively high. However, one of the reasons that the Wechsler has been so popular is that it allows for separate verbal and performance estimates. The organization of the subtests of the scale has made it possible for clinicians to undertake the analysis of the pattern of subtest scores for the same individual. This may be done because each subtest score can be expressed as a deviation from the mean score of the age group to which the subject belongs. Many clinicians have suggested that the particular pattern of scores for an individual provides information about his personality. A great deal of research has been done with pattern analysis and will be discussed in a later section.

The Wechsler-Bellevue Intelligence Scale, like the Binet, seems to be surrounded by a halo. There is no doubt that it has no present competition. It offers appropriate measurement of intelligence with adults only. Although there have been criticisms of the use of the standardization population which comes primarily from greater New York City, its sampling procedures are reasonably good. The limitations of testing people with language handicaps that applied to the Binet do not apply as much to the Wechsler, but the cultural and educational limitations do. The test score also reflects non intellective factors but is better designed to allow us to assess their operation.

Unlike the Binet, not only can it give a single index of mental ability, but the subtest arrangement allows us, with certain reservations, to obtain a profile of abilities. The most efficient method of doing this would require subtests which are not inter correlated and are highly reliable. Because Wechsler began with the notion of general intelligence, the subtests are highly intercorrelated and consequently subtest analysis with the Wechsler is highly inefficient. Moreover, some of the subtests themselves, particularly the performance tests, have rather low reliability for use in individual prediction. This is a point which will come up again in connection with the problem of diagnosis.

(a) VERBAL ITEMS

Information
What does rubber come from?
Comprehension
Why are people who are born deaf usually unable to talk?
Arithmetical teasoning
How many oranges can you buy for 36 cents if one oranges cost four cents?
Picture completion
Subject identifies what in missing

Digit span
Subject must repeat forward and backward series of digits ranging from three to nine.
Forward – 6,1,9,4,7,3,
Backward – 1,5,2,8,6
Similarities
In what way are the following things alike?
Orange – banana

(B) PERFORMANCE ITEMS

Picture completion
Subject identifies what is missing

ITEM 4

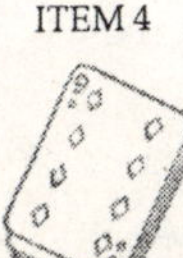

ITEM 15

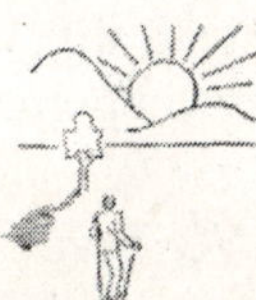

Picture arrangement
Subject must rearrange the picture to make a sensible sequence

ITEM 3

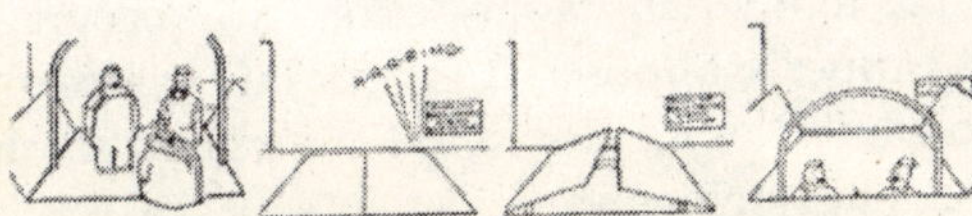

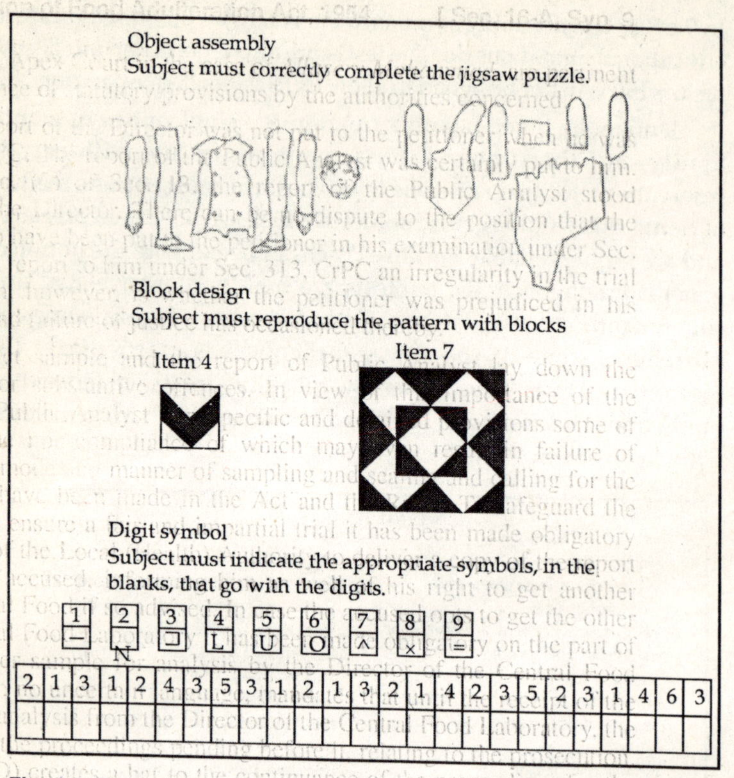

Fig. 4.2. Examples of Items on the Wechsler-Bellevue Intelligence Test.

The Wechsler does not suffer from the usual limitations of the IQ as it is defined on the Stanford-Binet. It has been criticized for the use' of the term IQ, but the statistic that Wechsler uses is a perfectly adequate one from a measurement point of view.

The empirical validity of the Wechsler is comparable to, if not better than, that of the Binet. We have pointed out that the typical correlations are by no means spectacular for individual prediction, but the Wechsler has yet to be excelled by any other measures of intelligence.

It is a valuable tool when its limitations are recognized and when the test is properly applied. It is certainly essential for the properly trained clinical psychologist to have a good command of the Wechsler-Bellevue Intelligence Scale.

Group Tests

The first group tests were arranged for adults, although later other age ranges were covered by this economical technique. We shall spend very little time with group tests. They are valuable assets to the psychologist because they enable him to obtain information cheaply and rapidly. However, given enough time, individually administered tests offer much more information to the clinician than do the group techniques. The main reason for this is the fact that in individual administration the situation of testing is so arranged that the clinical psychologist may make observations about the behavior of the individual in the testing experience. The argument for the use of group tests is entirely an economic one.

For subjects in the age range of about 7 to 15, a number of group verbal intelligence tests are available. Some cover the entire age range, and others are more limited. Some of these tests are: the Terman-McNemar Test of Mental Ability; the Otis tests and Thorndike 's CAVD scale. Some of the group nonverbal tests include: the Dearborn Group Tests (Series 1 is nonverbal, Series 2 contains some verbal material); the Chicago Non-Verbal Examination (by A. W. Brown, 1936); the Pintner Non-Language Series: Intermediate Test; the Non-Language MultiMental Test; the Progressive Matrices Test Culture-Free Test; and the Goodenough Drawing Test. A number of group tests not included in these lists contain verbal and nonverbal parts: the Kuhlmann-Anderson Intelligence Tests; the Pintner, Cunningham, and Durost Test ; the Dearborn Group Tests the California Tests of Mental Maturity and the Chicago Tests of Primary Mental Abilities.

For use with adults a number of group verbal and performance tests may be found. The Revised Army Alpha and the Revised Beta as well as the Pattern Perception Test are examples of these. There are other adult tests which are primarily verbal in character and which verge upon the aptitude type of test. The American Council on Education: Psychological Examination for College Freshmen, the Ohio State University Psychological Test, the College Entrance Board Examination: Scholastic Aptitude Test (annual versions not available), the Yale Educational Aptitude Battery, the Graduate Record Examination, and the Miller Analogies are examples of tests which are designed to predict success in higher education. The Army

General Classification Test used during the last war was concerned with the ability of men and women to learn military duties. While it was designed for this specific purpose, it also contained items which are typically found in standard intelligence tests.

As one can see, the number and variety of tests available which measure intellectual capacity is very large. The clinical psychologist must make correct decisions concerning the selection of the most appropriate test for his purposes. This requires not only a knowledge of testing principles but a familiarity with the tests available and with the sources of information about tests. His decision about which test or tests he should use will depend upon such varied considerations as what he wishes to measure, the subject's special limitations or particular characteristics, the reliability and validity of the test and its standardization, the amount of time available, and so on. The reader should consult textbooks which undertake to review these problems in order to gain the fullest perspective about the field of intelligence testing.

Tests of Achievement and Aptitude

We have pointed out in the last section the close relationship between many achievement tests and measures of intelligence. In fact, some of the intelligence tests contain items which measure some types of achievement, for example, amount of general information, solving arithmetic problems, etc. Achievement tests, like aptitude tests, are usually much more restricted in scope. They are often limited to single school subjects like arithmetic or history. They may include a battery of information tests in many school subjects. Or they may be designed to measure special verbal or motor skills.

Achievement tests may be used for a number of purposes: for grade placement; to assess the amount learned in a course of study; for personnel selection; and for diagnostic reasons, that is, to determine a pupil's strengths and weaknesses in various subjects so that corrective measures may be employed or guidance given.

To list all the achievement tests available would be of little value to the reader. Such a list would have to cover tests of reading ability, achievement in subjects ranging from elementary school to high school and college, and tests of special skills. For listings and discussions of these instruments, the reader is referred to textbooks by Cronbach, Freeman, Goodenough and Greene. Buros offers comprehensive listings and reviews of these tests.

What we have said about achievement tests applies in a large measure to the aptitude area as well. Prediction about the future acquisition of skills is useful primarily in personnel selection and in vocational guidance. The number of aptitudes that may be measured is almost unlimited. When we classify the aptitude tests, we find that there are not only a great many types but also a large number of tests of each aptitude as well. A full listing of them would include the following kinds of special aptitudes: mechanical, clerical, art, music, medicine, law, teaching, engineering, science, reading readiness, and aptitude for other special school subjects. Lists and discussions of these tests may be found in the same sources as for achievement tests.

Some aptitude test batteries attempt to measure basic verbal, motor, and perceptual talents as predictors of ability to learn other specialized skills. These measurements often enable the psychologist to make reasonable guesses concerning the general vocational areas in which a person could be successful. The individual with very poor spatial and perceptual abilities is likely to be a poor bet for training in mechanical engineering. On the other hand, he may have more of the talents necessary to be a successful lawyer. In the last war such test batteries were designed to select the best men for training as pilots, navigators, and bombardiers. Special psychomotor abilities were measured because of their predictive value in assessing potential ability in one of the Air Force training programs. Measures of reaction time, steadiness, complex coordination, and other abilities helped improve the efficiency of selection of these personnel. This is but one of the illustrations that may be used to point out the use of and types of tests which have been designed to measure special aptitudes.

Of course, the clinical significance of the aptitude tests rests primarily with their use in vocational guidance clinics. In the past 10 years the growth of vocational guidance activities has nearly paralleled the development of the standard psychological clinic. Guidance services have sprung up in universities as well as under the auspices of local departments of education and social service agencies. The Veterans Administration, which played so great a role in the expansion of the psychological clinic, also operates a large number of centers for vocational and educational advisement. In addition, in many cities vocational guidance services have become a fairly profitable kind of commercial enterprise.

All this activity rests upon the availability of the large number of tests of aptitude, achievement, and intelligence which are now available to vocational guidance workers. In many ways the services of these agencies have been valuable to large numbers of people when the application of vocational tests has been intelligent and when such tests have been carefully supplemented by interviews and data from other sources. On the other hand, the popularity of vocational guidance activities and the public belief in the infallibility of tests has led, in many instances, to abuses.

Many of these abuses have occurred because aptitude tests are much more accurate in the prediction of nonprofessional activities such as the skilled trades than in higher level jobs such as executive positions and professions. When the prediction must be made for lawyers, doctors, industrial vice-presidents, etc., the special aptitude tests are of minimal usefulness. Success in higher level activities depends so much on personality factors as well as upon specific talents that the tests of special aptitudes are most often inadequate. Of course, in the extreme cases of low or high capacity, it is often possible to say with confidence that the applicant is inadequate for the job. But more often it does not take a test to record the obvious fact that the person would be totally unsuited for the position. In using tests for selection and guidance many professional psychologists (knowingly or unknowingly) have abused the public confidence and have, perhaps, done irreparable damage to the profession to which they belong by making extravagant claims which cannot be substantiated.

The usefulness of aptitude tests for personnel selection and vocational guidance depends entirely upon the correlation of these tests with whatever skill or ultimate performance we are trying to predict. This correlation represents the validity of the test or test battery. The Air Force was able to make use of tests which had low validities because of the tremendous number of men who could be chosen for any job. It is often possible to use tests with low validities when the selection ratio is large, that is, when the proportion of men available for a job compared with the number of men needed is large. Low validity means that many mistakes will be made in prediction. People who would do very well at the job will be rejected. Moreover, many wrong choices will be made. However, in the military situation the entire enterprise was so vast that a large number of individual errors could be tolerated in the interest of the total program. It was actually possible to markedly reduce the number of failures in training through appropriate selection procedures.

Clinical predictions, in contrast with mass placement programs, are always made for one person, and we cannot as readily console ourselves with statistical averages. If the validity of a test used in vocational guidance or clinical diagnosis is low, then the probabilities that we will make an error in advisement are great. Our test results must always be evaluated with this in mind. The level of validity that we need for individual prediction with any degree of confidence is much higher than when we are predicting for a group. It is essential for us to recognize that faith in the mythical qualities of objective tests cannot be substituted for a thorough knowledge of their limitations and for the use of good sense in their interpretation.

5

Defects of Clinical Psychology

Introduction

The measurement of a person's intellectual capacity can be of great value to the clinical psychologist. It is often an essential part of the evaluation of a patient's personality. Information about the intellectual resources which an individual can bring to bear on his problems may make a considerable difference in the type of therapy undertaken with him. But in addition to this, the emotional problems of the person and the mechanisms by which he deals with them are often reflected in measurable ways in his intellectual performance. The individual's effectiveness and unique style in problem solving reflect the organization of his personality. Therefore, clinical psychologists have become interested in studying the intellectual processes as a means of obtaining information about the manner in which a person's emotional adjustment affects his performance. While perception, learning, reasoning, judgment, and all the other intellectual activities are interesting to the psychologist in themselves, to the clinician and personologist they offer excellent mediums for studying the individual's total personality in action. This is particularly true when it can be shown that the individual's intellectual functioning is defective. In such a case, not only can we use this information in making therapeutic decisions, but the nature of the intellectual defect may tell us something about the kind of emotional adjustment that the person is making.

In our historical survey of the field of clinical psychology, we noted that Esquirol was the first man to clearly differentiate simple lack of capacity from its loss as a consequence of disease. In the years which have followed, this distinction has remained with us. Various interpretations of the observations concerning defects of the intellect have been offered. To identify the impairment of mental functioning which resulted from physical or mental illness, terms like "dementia," "deterioration," and "regression" have been used. Because these terms are likely to convey implications concerning the theoretical explanation for the intellectual loss (which is poorly understood at the present time), Hunt and Cofer have preferred to use the term "psychological deficit." We like the expression intellectual deficit a little better, since it is possible to confuse psychological deficit with the affective disturbances which occur in mental diseases. However, both terms will do.

Throughout this chapter we shall use the expressions "intellectual deficit," "deficit," "impairment," and "loss" to refer to the harmful effects which psychological or physiological illness may have upon the intellectual processes.

Poor intellectual functioning may be spoken of as mental deficiency when the implication is drawn that the condition represents a lack of intellectual development rather than a loss due to disease. While the distinction is accepted in psychology and is certainly justifiable, it is really not clear-cut. It is not always a simple matter to determine whether an intellectually inadequate person represents a case of simple mental deficiency (that is, lack of development) or intellectual deficit (loss of powers which were once there). Moreover, some cases of mental deficiency may be etiologically closer to cases of intellectual deficit than to other cases of mental deficiency whose condition resulted from quite different causes. For example, it is believed that some mental deficiencies are caused by very early injuries to the central nervous system arising out of bacterial invasion. This deficiency appears to be essentially the same as the cases of deficit which develop much later (after the intellectual development has progressed to full maturity) as a consequence of the same bacterial invasion and similar damage to the central nervous system. Surely mental deficiency which results from infection during infancy is vastly different from the deficiency which appears to be hereditary in nature. Yet, for want of more information, the main distinction which is made between mental deficiency and intellectual deficit is that in the former case the intellectual development was retarded, while in the latter situation the intellectual functioning had once been "normal" and later, as a consequence of disease, was impaired or lost. In any case both conditions are types of pathological states with respect to intellectual functioning.

The emphasis in this chapter has been placed on the problem of intellectual deficit because we believe it is of greater potential importance to the clinician. It provides him with opportunities to understand the organization of intellectual and personality processes as well as with information to make better diagnostic formulations about a particular patient's mental illness. Most of this chapter will be concerned with the theoretical and practical problems of understanding and measuring intellectual deficit. However, since it is an important related problem which is difficult to untangle from the question of deficit, we shall first have some things to say about mental deficiency.

Mental Deficiency

The earliest psychological clinics owed their existence, in part, to the great interest in mental deficiency in the early 1900's. The later clinics, particularly as they developed around 1930, were much less dominated by the consideration of the problem child. Relative to the tremendous expansion of clinical interest and facilities, there appeared to be a lessening of interest in the problems of mental deficiency. The development of the Veterans Administration mental hygiene organization following the last war increased the percentage of psychological clinics devoted mainly to adult problems. There appears to be, however, some recent upsurge in activity with children and some renewed interest in mental deficiency. There is no doubt that some of the most fascinating theoretical and practical problems may be found in this area. Space should be devoted, therefore, to some of these problems. We cannot attempt to present a complete account of considerations which arise out of the study of mental deficiency.

A great many forms of behavior have been classed under the term mental deficiency. But the practical question of who is mentally deficient and who is not continues to confront us. The effectiveness of our research in this area depends upon the resolution of the problem of identifying properly and consistently what it means to be mentally deficient. This will also determine the treatment of patients who are mentally deficient. Classification, etiology, and measurement are all interrelated and basic problems. We shall discuss the main considerations in the study of these problems in the sections which follow.

Measurement: What we really are concerned with in the case of measurement is, "Who is mentally deficient?" Most people would answer this question by referring to our intelligence tests. Many clinicians have continued to use the IQ or some comparable measure as the major and often only indication of the diagnosis of mental deficiency.

The problem is still more complicated. There are many ways of getting the same IQ. The kinds of intellectual strengths and weaknesses which make up the total score may vary greatly between individuals with the same IQ. The total measure therefore does not tell us very well what the individual can and cannot do.

Furthermore, some people think of intelligence in terms of social adaptiveness. There is nothing wrong with this, nor is it necessarily better than relating it to our tests. People with high academic degrees may behave very foolishly in social situations. Two people with the same IQ, both mentally deficient in these terms, may differ greatly in social adaptiveness. These differences, in fact, may be so great that one such person may have to be institutionalized while the other is gainfully employed and makes a reasonably acceptable citizen. The question of which people are mentally deficient is, therefore, not a simple one and cannot be decided by the IQ alone.

Many suggestions have been made concerning what kinds of criteria should be used in identifying a mentally deficient individual. The British have tended to lean toward the use of some estimate of social adequacy, while Americans have tended to go overboard for the IQ. Representing the former view is Tredgold, who goes so far in this direction that he would classify some persons having an average IQ as mentally deficient because they have failed to care for themselves adequately in the community. The best example of the advocate of more inclusive criteria of mental deficiency in this country is Doll. Doll has repeatedly emphasized the inadequacy of the IQ as a satisfactory criterion. His own criteria include subnormal test intelligence, social incompetence, arrested development rather than retrogression (deficit), presence of the defect at maturity, constitutional origin, and incurability. One may question the inclusion of many of Doll's criteria which he maintains must be present for a conclusive diagnosis of mental deficiency. Some of them are not too practical for the clinic, since it takes a long time to assess the curability of mental deficiency. Moreover, the constitutional decision can rarely be positive. To implement the evaluation of social competence, Doll introduced a test of social maturity which has gained wide acceptance in recent years. This test will be described in a later chapter on personality measurement. By interviewing someone in close touch with the child in question, the scale may be used to obtain evidence of linguistic, social, and motor development and relate this to norms for each particular age level from infancy to adulthood.

The chief problem in the application of the social-competency criterion in the diagnosis of mental deficiency is the vagueness and subjectivity involved in this kind of evaluation. How do we judge the social inadequacy? In what kinds of social functions should we look for competence and incompetence? Doll has undoubtedly helped matters in a practical sense with the social-maturity scale. But more must be learned about which intellectual functions are associated with different kinds of adjustments so that they may be used diagnostically and prognostically.

Interest among psychologists in measurement other than the global IQ is a step in the right direction. Jastak recently criticized the use of the social and statistical criteria of mental deficiency and has offered an additional criterion. He points out that we never really measure capacity, although this is what we may be trying to estimate. Actually we are measuring the level of performance that a person has achieved, and this may be far below his maximum altitude. Jastak suggests that the best estimate of maximum level or capacity is the function which yields the highest score. He is suggesting a special use of scatter analysis which is a diagnostic technique we shall discuss later in connection with intellectual deficit. An individual with an IQ which is statistically at the feeble-minded level, but who achieves some subtest scores at or near normal, is not feeble-minded according to Jastak.

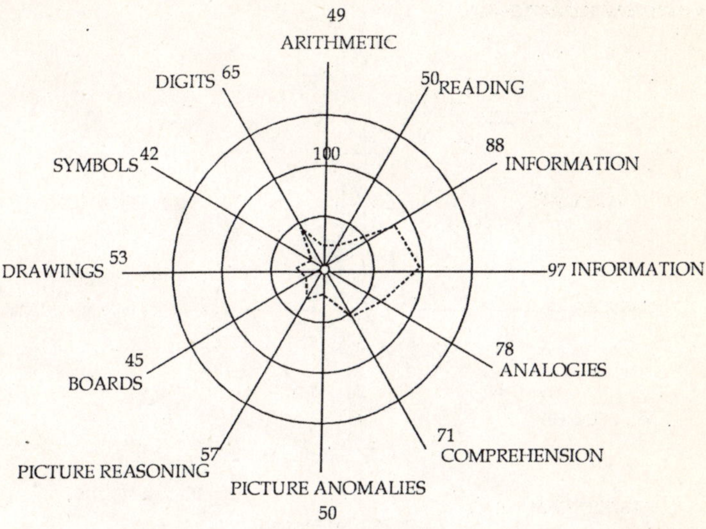

Fig. 5.1. Test Results of Clinic Case A on Psychometric Patterns. Psychiatric Diagnosis: Schizoid Personality in Person of Average Intelligence.

We must seek other explanations of his poor performance, perhaps in emotional or motivational factors. He presents a number of test profiles of patients with identical IQ's but markedly different patterns and maximal levels. They are reproduced here in Figure. 3.

Jastak maintains that cases that are socially or economically successful are really not feeble-minded (this is part of his definition of mental deficiency) and that the use of his criterion would eliminate the inconsistency of finding patients who were diagnosed feeble-minded who later became economically and socially self-sustaining. His arguments are cogent, but the data are at present unavailable which would indicate whether or not such a technique would in reality be superior to what is suggested by Doll and would, indeed, enable the training schools to concentrate on the appropriate patients.

Classification . Classification is the first and most primitive step in the scientific process. It involves grouping our observations in terms of their common elements. Our earliest divisions into classes usually must be revised over and over again because, as we learn more about the phenomena under observation, we discover that we must change the basis of classification in order to bring it in line with new information.

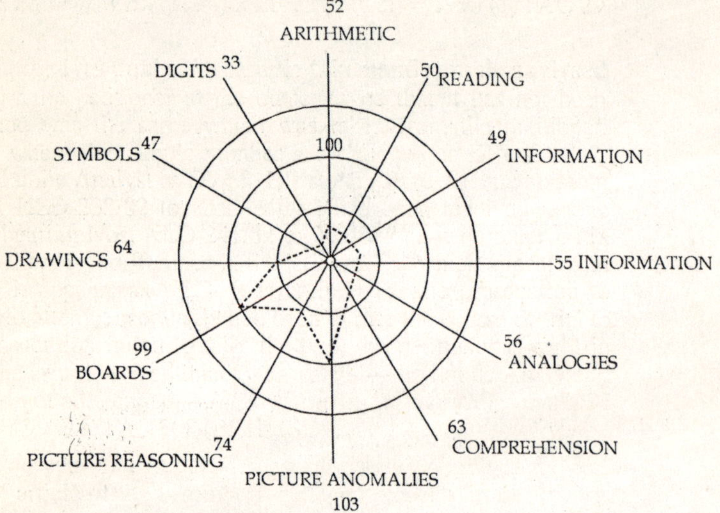

Fig. 5.2. Test Results of Clinic Case B on Psychometric Patterns. Psychiatric Diagnosis: Psychopathic Personality in a Person of Average Intelligence.

If we examine all the known varieties of mental deficiency, we notice that we can identify a group in which defective intelligence seems to be mild, to run in the family, and which appears to have no complications like brain injury, disease, or other characteristics which might be presumed to be the causal conditions of the defect. Studies of these cases have suggested that a hereditary factor could be responsible for the mental inadequacy. This group of cases has been identified in a number of ways by workers in this area. Sarason has called them the "garden-variety" of mental defective. Others such as Lewis have called this group the "endogenous" mental deficiencies. Strauss has used the term "subcultural." There has been no agreement concerning the real etiological features of this class, and many theorists are still arguing the nature-nurture question. In these cases the role of physiological, genetic, and motivational factors is difficult to parcel out.

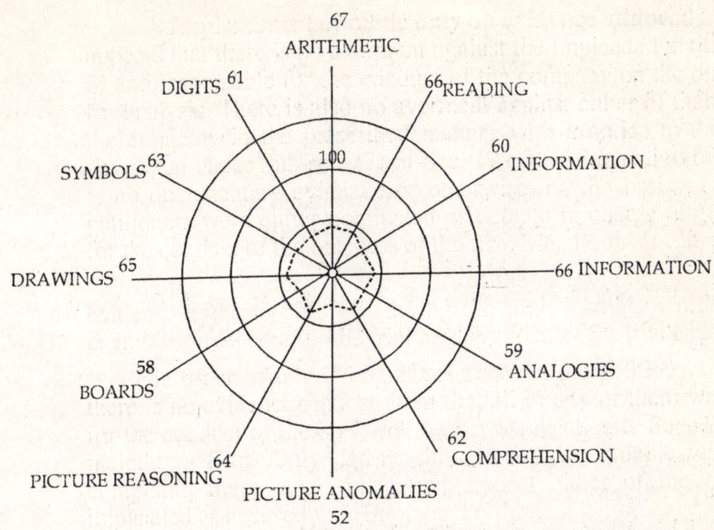

Fig. 5.3. Test Results of Clinic Case C on Psychometric Patterns. Psychiatric Diagnosis: Inherent Mental Deficiency, Moron Level, in a Person of Adaptable Personality.

Poor intellectual performance has also been found in a large number of other types of settings. This symptom may be found among the psychoses, in cases with the presence of organic disease, metabolic disorders, congenital injuries, and special hereditary defects. Most modern-day thinking makes use of a dichotomous classification, with the garden-variety mental defective (considered by some as the only true feeble-minded group) on the one hand and all the other types of mental deficiencies lumped into another group and further subdivided in terms of what is thought to be their specific etiology.

Most of the classification systems are the most convenient descriptive ways of grouping cases and reflect present-day ignorance concerning the nature of the mental processes. For example, when Tredgold divided mental deficiency into four classes, amentia due to inheritance, amentia due to environment, amentia due to both inheritance and environment, and amentia without discoverable cause, he was groping in the dark. Such a division is arbitrary and does not fit into any real knowledge concerning the nature of mental defects. Nor is it possible at the present time to make any well grounded diagnosis for these classes.

It is quite probable that the mental deficiencies hang together only in the most superficial sense and that the basis of the garden-variety type is entirely different from cases, described by Jastak and others, who perform some tasks at an average level or higher. Moreover, these two forms of mental deficiency may have little direct relation to cases with such physiological conditions as metabolic disorders. If this is true, then any classification based upon similarities in symptomatology must eventually be revised when we know more about the nature of intellectual behavior.

From the clinician's point of view, the classification would be of value at the moment if it allowed him to make the proper decisions concerning what should be done with each group. Little is known along these lines. What should be done with the garden-variety type of defective is not agreed upon. Doll maintains that the group he calls feeble-minded cannot be treated effectively, since there is no chance of the development of social competency. Some kinds of defectives he believes can be helped. Jastak, who would identify the former feeble-minded group as those with low intellectual performance on all tests and subtests (low scatter), appears to agree that the truly feeble-minded are never successfully able to manage their affairs adequately in spite of any training methods. If this were true and this group could be reliably identified, the course of action that should be taken would certainly be different from that used with those mentally deficient individuals whose defect is largely a function of motivational or emotional variables. At the present, resolution of this difficulty remains one of the crucial problems in the field of mental deficiency. Research which will clarify the potentialities of the various classes of mentally deficient people is lacking, has been inadequate, or has produced controversial results.

Etiology . While all the problems we have discussed are interwoven with the question of etiology, a few words might be said about this problem specifically. While many cases of mental deficiency have been associated with some metabolic condition, infection, or neurological damage, and seem to be the result of these conditions, the exact nature of the effects of these causal agents is not known in any instance. We can mention only some of these conditions here.

Mental deficiency has been found, on rare occasions, to be associated with the incomplete oxidation of an amino acid, phenylalanine. In these cases phenylpyruvic acid is found excreted in the urine. The condition appears to be genetically determined. The work of Penrose, Jervis and others has thrown some light on this condition. A number of organic conditions seem to be associated with the symptoms of mental deficiency. For example, epilepsy has been found associated with both slight and severe mental impairment. Infections of the nervous system such as meningitis, encephalitis, and congenital syphilis appear under some circumstances to produce losses in mental functioning. Cranial deformities and pressure by the cerebrospinal fluid are another source. German measles in pregnancy (especially early in pregnancy) has been associated with mongolism, and irradiation with X rays during pregnancy has also been thought of as an etiological factor in some mental deficiencies. Metabolic disorders such as cretinism are also known to produce permanent damage if not checked early. But exactly how these conditions work to produce the mental defects is not clear, although the assumption has been that irreversible change or destruction of nervous tissue is the common cause. As we have noted, some mental deficiencies have been thought to be primarily inherited. For more detailed accounts and a bibliography of these etiological factors the reader is referred to Sarason. The state of medical knowledge in this area is quite limited.

The causes and effects of some of these mental-deficiency syndromes are better understood than others, although in any case their precise influence on the intellectual processes is nowhere near known. For example, it is known that mental deficiency may be associated with meningitis, probably through the destruction of brain tissues. However, the majority of people who have had meningitis show no intellectual impairment that can be measured, even though they may show physical disabilities. It is reasonable to attribute this to differences in the tissues which are damaged by the disease, but we do not know which tissues are important and how this deficiency is related to many of the other conditions. The same thing may be said about hydrocephaly and syphilis, both of which produce destruction of brain tissue. Moreover, although cretinism is a metabolic disorder resulting in intellectual deficiency, the exact nature of the effect of this disease on the nervous system remains to be discovered.

There is no doubt that severe mental illness may produce what appears to be deficiency of intellectual performance. It is not clear how mental illness operates to produce this effect. In some ways the question grows out of the arbitrary division of psychological processes into cognitive, motivational, and affective. There can be little doubt that what we measure in performance is not solely an intellectual thing but reflects motivational and emotional influence. In fact, if we thought of performance as an expression of the total personality of the individual, we might consider at least some cases of defective intelligence as a reflection of a defective personality. Even if capacity were a fixed physiological variable, performance is all we ever observe, and it is certainly a function of personality variables.

In any event, we are left with huge problems in the area of mental deficiency. The basic ones are: (1) What conditions produce the different types of mental-deficiency syndromes? (2) What are the mechanisms of their effect upon the intellectual processes? (3) What are the potential outcomes of each of the syndromes, and what treatment or disposition is indicated for them? (4) What kinds of measuring devices and indices can be used to differentiate the different types? And finally, (5) What is the real nature of the processes we call intellectual, and how do these processes relate to the practical problems of adjustment to the environment?

Intellectual Deficit

There are a large number of observational and experimental studies in this field. If the reader wishes a fuller presentation of the research up to 1944, the Hunt and Cofer article previously cited will furnish an excellent beginning. We shall attempt to discuss only the highlights in the theoretical and practical side of the study of psychological deficit.

The large variety of researches into deficit have arisen from a great number of different frames of reference and have been undertaken for various purposes. In many instances, comparison of the results cannot be made properly because different functions have been measured or different tests used. The methods used have differed so greatly that comparison of the studies becomes, in many instances, impossible.

The general study of intellectual impairment is of great importance for three main reasons. The research findings should be of help in our understanding of the various clinical disorders. They should also throw some light on the nature of intellectual functioning. Moreover, in the practical clinical situation, the data could be applied to the study of the psychological status of the individual patient. In the latter instance, the measurement of the pattern of intellectual functioning in a particular patient becomes part of the diagnostic picture. In the sections that follow we shall first discuss the theoretical interpretations of the findings on deficit, indicate the kinds of functions measured, and describe the techniques of measurement.

Theoretical Explanations of Deficit: A number of theoretical explanations of a fairly unsystematic sort have been offered by different psychologists to account for deficit behavior. Because so little is really known about this question, it will not pay us to do more than merely mention the main points of view that may be expressed by people who attempt to interpret the observations. We must also point out that the kinds of functions measured in experiments on deficit represent such a hodgepodge that it may be reasonable to speak of many kinds of deficits. One theoretical approach may make better sense when considered in connection with one kind of disorder than with another.

Generally speaking, workers in this field have preferred to think of intellectual deficit in one of two ways. Some have attempted to approach the problem on a psychological level, and others have looked for explanations from a physiological point of view. Little real success has been obtained with either approach up to the present.

Psychological Views: In the psychological approach, many of the so-called explanations are little more than descriptive statements. The most cogent psychological way of thinking of intellectual deficit in the functional psychoses and psychoneuroses appears to us to be a motivational viewpoint. Observation of schizophrenic patients, for example, strongly suggests that failure or impairment in cognitive functions does not really represent loss of capacity in those areas but lack of motivation to sustain attention to the task or conflicting motives associated with psychological threat. This point of view is all the more impressive with the observation that, with more adequate rapport and some coaxing, the previously failing schizophrenic patient may improve his performance greatly. The motivational view includes the possibility that the functional disorder is a mechanism of adjustment of some kind which is adopted when other mechanisms fail. The patient's defense against threat is to restrict his sphere of responsiveness so that it appears to the observer that he has lost his capacity for certain functions that were previously intact. One instance of this kind of defense is the condition known to child psychologists as "pseudo-feeble-mindedness." In this case a child with normal intellectual capacity performs at the level of the feeble-minded child because of emotional withdrawal from competition and social threat. With therapeutic attention he may improve radically.

Physiological View: Proponents of the physiological approach to deficit have, in the past, spoken of cerebral pathology or endocrine disorders as the important features to look for. The mental disorders have been thought by some to be related to heredity, body type, and more recently, to metabolic functions. Some recent arguments in support of the metabolic view may be found in the work of Hoagland. Others have been struck by the similarity of the deficit between patients with organic brain pathology and the schizophrenias, believing that this indicates a common organic pathology. Few of these leads have borne real fruit at the present time. Whether it will be more profitable in the long run to investigate deficit through the behavioral frame of reference or the physiological one is not clear at our present stage of progress. Neither approach has effectively dealt with the problem of the nature of intellectual deficit. At best, we have a large quantity of unsystematic observations and theory which suffer mostly from a lack of completely satisfactory methodology.

Types of Functions Measured: A wide variety of cognitive functions has been studied by researches into intellectual deficit. Nearly all conceivable kinds of measures have been made with most of the standard types of tools for the study of intellectual capacity. The most common of these types of measures include mental age and IQ scores, tests of vocabulary, reasoning, immediate memory, judgment, and a large group of other similar and related processes. In addition to these more typical measures, psychologists have studied receptive processes which include sensory thresholds and perceptual behavior. The sensory studies, most of which have tended to be weak on technique, have not yielded much by way of dependable differences between various types of patients and non patients. The perceptual studies, on the other hand, have discovered impairment of functioning in copying geometric designs on the part of schizophrenics, changes in the figure-ground fluctuations of manic-depressives, and a number of other deficits for these and other patient groups. In the past few years, interest in the apparent relationships between motivations and perceptual behavior has led to a renewed attack on the perceptual process in various psychological disturbances. For a long time there has been great interest in the perceptual processes in patients who have some kind of organic brain damage.

A wide variety of response processes has also been investigated with the expectation of coming up with significant relationships between different disorders and the cognitive functions measured. Researchers have studied functions such as response times of various types (simple, complex, verbal, motor), word association, memory, language and thought, conditioning, and emotional behavior. Many of these investigations have borne interesting fruit. Little agreement will be found, however, concerning the way in which many of the observations should be interpreted. The field is now handicapped because of methodological difficulties and the lack of any systematic theory concerning the real nature of the psychological changes which seem to occur in some mental disorders.

Techniques of Measurement: The concept of intellectual deficit assumes a temporary or permanent loss or impairment of some functions which had previously been present or at a higher level. The technically ideal method of demonstrating the presence of deficit would therefore require some measure of these functions before the disorder intervened and produced the impairment. This could then be compared with measurements during or following the disorder. Because of the lack of these premorbid scores in patients with mental disorders, all the techniques for the measurement of deficit have depended upon various ways of estimating what the intellectual status of the patient was before the onset of the present condition. The existence of increasingly complete records on large numbers of men in the military service and in the public-school systems may make it possible in the future to use this more desirable approach of having premorbid measures. Rapaport and Webb have recently demonstrated deficit by the use of premorbid intelligence tests (measured in high school). However, lack of control cases reduces the usefulness of these data.

Even this technique often offers hazards: We can never be sure that, when we first tested these people, they were not then suffering from some degree of deficit. The best illustration of this problem may be found in some of the recent studies of the effect of electric shock or brain surgery on the intellectual functions. Preoperative measures were available in this instance, but the assumption that these measures were obtained on psychologically intact organisms could not safely be made. In most instances, the patients operated upon or shocked were badly deteriorated during the time of the first testing or were in such severe pain (as in the case of incurable cancers) that no satisfactory estimates of original intellectual level were possible. Moreover, the question of how sensitive our tests are to slight and even moderate impairment always plagues us.

In place of the use of premorbid measures, there have been devised two major ways of studying intellectual deficit. The first approach is entirely normative in nature, that is, it makes use of central tendencies in the functions to be measured among various diagnostic groups. We have called this the "group-comparison technique." The second general technique emphasizes an intra individual analysis. We have called this the "subtest-pattern technique." The latter approach studies the pattern of performance on different functions within a patient and refers this pattern to norms which have been established for various types of disturbances. Let us examine how these procedures work and the problems that arise in their use.

Group-comparison Technique: Properly used, this procedure requires the selection of a group of patients which is homogeneous with respect to kind of disorder and compares it with another group, usually normal, which is similar in certain important variables. The matching on the relevant variables may be done on a group basis. For example, the selection of the two groups is made so that such variables as age, education, cultural background, and any other factors which must be controlled are equivalent for both groups. On the other hand, the matching may be done by individuals, that is, for every patient a control is selected who is comparable in all the important respects. The patient group may be compared with the controls in such measures as mental age, IQ, or in any of the intellectual, sensory, perceptual, or response functions. Differences in average performance in favor of the control population are interpreted as suggesting the presence of deficit in the other group. The control group is therefore used as a standard to estimate the premorbid level of the patient group.

In both the group and individual matching procedures, the comparison depends upon the equivalence of both groups with respect to the appropriate variables. The danger in the use of these procedures lies mainly in compromising with these controls out of necessity and ignoring variables because they are thought to be unimportant. A perfect match is virtually impossible even with the greatest care. Consequently, we frequently have to assume that differences between controls and experimental subjects are insignificant, irrelevant, or are randomized by the use of as large a sample as possible. These are often dangerous assumptions.

A large number of studies of this type have been attempted. It is not possible to review them here. Many of them have been discussed by Hunt and Cofer. Other reviews may be found in Hunt, Rouvroy, Wechsler, Kendig and Richmond, Roe and Shakow and Brody. Examination of them shows that the studies varied greatly with respect to the types of measures employed and the adequacy of the controls used. The great disagreement that is found among the various studies can probably be laid to this lack of controls, differences in the functions measured, sampling, and differences in the testing techniques used.

From this work certain conclusions appear to be reasonable at least on a tentative basis. There tends to be agreement that some degree of deficit, using standard intelligence tests, is found in nearly all the disorders with the possible exception of the psychoneurotics and patients following brain surgery or convulsive therapy. The deficit is most marked in the organic psychoses. Certain types of tests do not appear to suffer as much loss as others. For example, information and vocabulary hold up well under the disease process, while tests requiring conceptual thinking, speed, and sustained associative thinking show losses. The more complex or difficult the function measured, the greater the degree of deficit appears to be.

The general failure to employ adequate sampling, to properly match groups, to measure comparable functions, and to use comparable techniques has left the normative study of psychological deficit in a fairly inadequate state. There is still a need for this type of study.

Probably more crucial than any other single question is the problem of the adequacy of our current tests. Most of them were not designed for the purpose of measuring deficit. Many are not too reliable. Moreover, there is the great problem of identifying the functions that we are really measuring. As long as we do not know the interrelationships between our tests, the nature of cognitive processes, and the role of emotional and motivational factors in performance, we can do little more than to haphazardly describe the strengths and weaknesses of various diagnostic groups. Even at that, we fall into the difficulty of using a diagnostic scheme that is little more than a rough classification by symptoms and which is coming in for more and more criticism among clinical psychologists and psychiatrists at the present time. Our present labeling devices for disease syndromes and tests seem to have led us into a blind alley.

Subtest-Pattern Technique: This technique of studying deficit uses the pattern of scores within the record of a single patient to estimate his premorbid level. It depends upon the now common observations that some functions like vocabulary hold up (or do not show much loss) in mental disturbances while others show considerable impairment. By comparing the degree of deviation of test scores which usually show loss in mental illness from those which generally hold up, a diagnostic statement may be made about the patient. The actual pattern of subtest scores may be analyzed, or a simple measure of the degree of scatter may be obtained to show the spread of subtest scores. Remember that while this is an intra individual measure, that is, it deals with the variation of different performances of the same person, the interpretation of such patterns depends on its comparison with the pattern of some normative group. We can say nothing about a particular patient's pattern unless we know what is found in other patients or groups of people with or without the symptoms of illness.

Subtest-pattern analysis appears to have obtained its impetus from some work by Wells, although the technique has even earlier roots in connection with the problem of delinquency. In 1930, Babcock developed a workable method of measuring psychological deficit, employing vocabulary as an estimate of original intellectual capacity. Babcock used as her measures of loss, tests of new learning, motor efficiency, immediate memory, and a number of other functions which were readily impaired in the mental disorders. In standardizing her technique, she administered these tests along with the Terman Vocabulary list to a group of "normal" adults. She then adjusted the scores on vocabulary so that the normal-group average was the same as on the rest of the battery of tests. In other words, the average difference for the group between scores on the vocabulary test and each other test was set at zero. Testing a sample of paretics, she found differences in efficiency scores which supported the notion that patients with organic brain damage would show a characteristic loss of efficiency in certain functions, namely, motor skills and new learning. Later a similar finding was demonstrated with schizophrenic patients. These tests have since been revised for clinical use.

With this beginning, the diagnostic use of differential patterns and the construction of new instruments for this special kind of measurement became a major activity of clinical psychologists. The original Babcock technique, which employed vocabulary as the best estimate of original capacity, was extended to the use of other measures like information, which were thought to "hold up" in the mental diseases. Despite the difficulties with the use of this technique with our present instruments, the Babcock approach has been exceedingly popular and useful to the clinician. The literature on the subject has become voluminous and rather controversial.

A simpler form of subtest-pattern analysis consists of a measure of the degree of scatter of the subtests in an individual test record. In the analysis of subtest patterns, we are interested in the kinds of tests selectively failed by the patient. In the scatter analysis the main interest is in some measure of the degree of spread of the subtest scores without reference to which items show extremely high-level performance and which result in exceptionally poor attainment.

There are many different kinds of scatter analyses depending for the most part upon the test which is used. We shall have occasion to briefly describe some of these techniques as they apply to some of the tests such as the Stanford-Binet and the Wechsler-Bellevue. All the techniques involve some variation of the basic theme of the degree of deviation in subtest scores from some established level or reference point. The use of scatter measures assumes that large amounts of scatter are indicative of emotional disturbances. The more the scatter, the greater the disturbance is presumed to exist. The individual is performing erratically, at a high level in some functions, with impairment in others. The procedure has been used by many clinicians to make decisions concerning whether a child is feeble-minded or suffering from an emotional disorder.

Some workers like Jastak, Kinder, Kinder and Hamlin, Bijou and others have argued that large scatter (in which a child with a subnormal intelligence performs well above the feeble-minded level on one or more subtests and below in others) may contraindicate a simple feeble-minded diagnosis. Some investigations have upheld the assumption on which scatter analysis rests, showing larger scatter in the performances of psychotic patients than in normal or simply feeble-minded children. Others like Harris and Shakow and Kendig and Richmond have obtained negative results when better controls were introduced. At the present time the use of scatter analysis as a sole criterion of anything appears to be of very doubtful validity. Many clinicians believe that scatter analysis is diagnostically useful, and it continues as a frequently practiced technique. Undoubtedly the construction of the Wechsler-Bellevue Scale is superior to the Stanford-Binet for this purpose, although its use is limited to adults. However, it is difficult to see how simple scatter analysis with present-day instruments and in the absence of validated pattern analysis can ever be more than a rough screening technique to encourage the clinician to look a little further.

Qualitative Observations: In addition to the study of quantitative patterns and scatter analysis, the performance of the individual may be examined from another point of view. Aspects of the performance such as response times, rate of response, amount of productivity, form of the response, projective content, and the attitudes and emotions that the individual displays to the testing itself or to certain parts of the testing may produce information which is of great importance in diagnostic evaluation. Since this approach provides a broader opportunity to study the personality of the individual, we shall discuss it in our later chapter on projective techniques. However, it should be pointed out here that any individual situation provides some opportunity for the subject to perform in qualitative ways which distinguish him as a unique individual. These features often provide the clinical psychologist with important cues concerning the personality dynamics.

Tests of Deficit: In this section we shall discuss the main diagnostic psychological tests on which the group-comparison and the subtest-pattern techniques of deficit measurement have been applied. In addition, we shall describe a group of instruments which were specifically designed for the measurement of certain kinds of psychological deficit. In the former category, we have included the Stanford-Binet and the Wechsler-Bellevue. The latter class comprises the Babcock, the Shipley-Hartford, the Hunt-Minnesota, and the special concept tests.

Stanford-Binet: The pattern-analysis technique has, on occasion, been used with the Stanford-Binet Intelligence Test. Various attempts have been made at grouping the subtests into clinically determined clusters which appear to measure the same functions. For example, visual perception, memory span, word knowledge, reasoning, and other groupings have been established on the basis of appearance and clinical intuition. In this way the intellectual strengths and weaknesses of any child may be studied. This pattern may then be compared with normative data for various clinical groups. Unfortunately, the normative data available are not entirely satisfactory for this purpose, and any attempt at this time to follow such a procedure is hazardous. Moreover, the technique of grouping by clinical intuition when factorial techniques are available has been under considerable fire in recent years.

Despite considerable uncertainty about its validity, the special technique of scatter analysis with the Binet has continued to be used. Harris and Shakow have classified measures of scatter on the Binet into three types: (1) Counting the number of years or age levels over which successes and failures are found. An example might help: One child with a mental age of 9 years may miss subtests as far down as the 5-year level and pass an item at year 12. Another child with the same mental age may have a range which runs from 7 years to 10. The former child has a degree of scatter which is well beyond the typical finding for most normal children and, therefore, to the clinician using this technique is suspect with regard to emotional disturbance and deficit. (2) Counting the number of months' credit which are earned above and below the basal year (the first year in which there are no subtest failures). (3) Applying some formula which takes both range and credits into account and weighting them in terms of their distance from the mental age level. The first method is the simplest to apply and understand.

Wechsler-Bellevue: In using the technique of pattern analysis the Bellevue has certain advantages over the Stanford-Binet. The items are grouped (according to the functions which they are supposed to measure) into 11 subtests, with norms and standard scores for each one.

The number of studies which have been performed with pattern analysis on the Wechsler-Bellevue is very large. Most of them deal with the ability to make differential diagnoses by matching the subtest pattern with normative data. Most of these attempts have been disappointing because of frequent disagreement between studies concerning what kind of patterns are to be found in the various types of disorders. Some general agreement may be found, however. For example, most studies agree that schizophrenics do better with the information and comprehension subtests than with object assembly and digit symbol.

The trouble in the area lies partly in the fact that there is so much overlap between diagnostic groups. The use of hospital diagnoses as criteria of validity is most dangerous in view of the lack of agreement between and even within hospital staffs and the doubtful meaning that a diagnostic label carries. The reliabilities of the subtests are also too low in many instances to serve the function of individual prediction.

A number of quantitative indexes have been devised which are intended to differentiate between one or another diagnostic group. For example, Rabin devised a schizophrenic index which consists of the ratio of the sum of the scores on information, comprehension, and block design (which are expected to hold up in schizophrenia) to the summated scores on the digit-symbol, object-assembly, and similarities tests. This has failed to materialize as a valid measure.

Wechsler himself devised what he called a "deterioration quotient" for evaluating the approximate amount of impairment of intellectual functioning in advancing age. Certain tests are presumed to hold up, that is, not decline with age and mental illness, while others do decline. The "hold" tests are information, comprehension, object assembly, picture completion, and vocabulary. Those tests which are believed to decline are digit span, arithmetic, digit symbol, block design, similarities, and picture arrangement. In calculating the index, the total of "don't-hold" scores is subtracted from the "hold" scores and divided by the total of the "hold" scores. The index derived represents, for Wechsler, the percentage of deterioration. This figure is then corrected for whatever loss is expected or normal at the particular age level of the patient, so that the resulting percentage is the extent of loss in excess of expected loss for that age group.

This method has also proved disappointing. Its usefulness probably lies in cases where impairment is extreme. In a study by Fox and Birren, Wechsler 's index failed to show any agreement with similar measures derived from the Babcock test. A large proportion of the studies of subtest patterns with schizophrenic patients has produced negative or questionable results. As Wittenborn has pointed out, even in studies with favorable results, simply inspecting the records for a few conspicuous instances of subtest failure and success would have been as valuable as the more elaborate pattern analyses. At the present time the use of pattern analysis is highly questionable because of conflicting evidence, standardization inadequacies, and the lack of satisfactory reliability among the various subtests. There is no doubt that the situation could be vastly improved. Clinicians are still trying. Recently Copple devised a somewhat different index which he calls a score of "senescent decline." Few data are as yet available to evaluate this attempt at providing an index of deficit from the Wechsler-Bellevue Scale.

As in the case with the Stanford-Binet, the Bellevue may also be used for scatter analysis as well as pattern analysis. There are several types of techniques available based on different reference points from which the scatter is calculated. In keeping with the observation that vocabulary does not show much loss, one measure of scatter makes use of the differences between the various subtest scores and the score obtained on vocabulary. In addition, the mean of the subtests may be used as the reference point and the deviation of each subtest taken from it. The mean used may be taken from the entire group of subtests, or it may be the performance mean (with deviations obtained for the performance subtests independently) or the mean of the verbal subtests. Finally, pairs of subtests may be compared to determine how much the subject's functioning in one area deviates from that in another.

The fact that the weighted scores on the Wechsler-Bellevue are a form of standard score makes such a procedure possible. However, low subtest reliability makes the technique statistically dangerous. As in the case of the Binet, this scatter technique, without pattern analysis, could be useful only as a rough screening device to alert the clinician to take a more careful look at the patient's functioning.

Babcock Test: As we have noted earlier, the Babcock test was specifically devised to measure intellectual impairment in individual patients suffering from various forms of mental and organic disturbances. It was originally used with practices and then with schizophrenics and other clinical groups. The test uses vocabulary as the reference point from which to study loss in efficiency in other functions like new learning, motor skills, immediate memory, and information.

The subtests have been arranged into a number of groups. These groups have been called by Babcock: easy tests (common information), learning, repetition, motor, easy continuous, and initial learning. The score for each group is the average of the subtests in it. The total average of all the groups combined is called the "efficiency score." The important estimate of the degree of impairment has been given the term "the efficiency index" by Babcock. This is obtained by converting the vocabulary score on the Terman Vocabulary Test into a vocabulary age. On the basis of this vocabulary age, the expected average level of performance on the groups of subtests is estimated using data from a normal population. The obtained group scores are averaged to find the efficiency score. Subtracting the expected average score from the obtained efficiency score yields the efficiency index. This index may be either positive or negative and in the negative direction indicates the degree of intellectual impairment. If the efficiency index is positive, there is presumed to be evidence of good functioning. The size of the negative index appears to be positively related to the degree of impairment.

Some clinical psychologists have attempted to use the pattern of subtest performance on the Babcock test for differential diagnosis. They have attempted to find patterns which are characteristic of the various psychiatric classes as has been done with the Wechsler-Bellevue. The general assumptions behind the use of the Babcock test of efficiency are basically the same as in the case of the scatter-analysis technique with the Binet and Wechsler. However, overlapping of profiles and unreliability have made this procedure relatively unrewarding up to the present, just as we have found to be the case with the Wechsler-Bellevue.

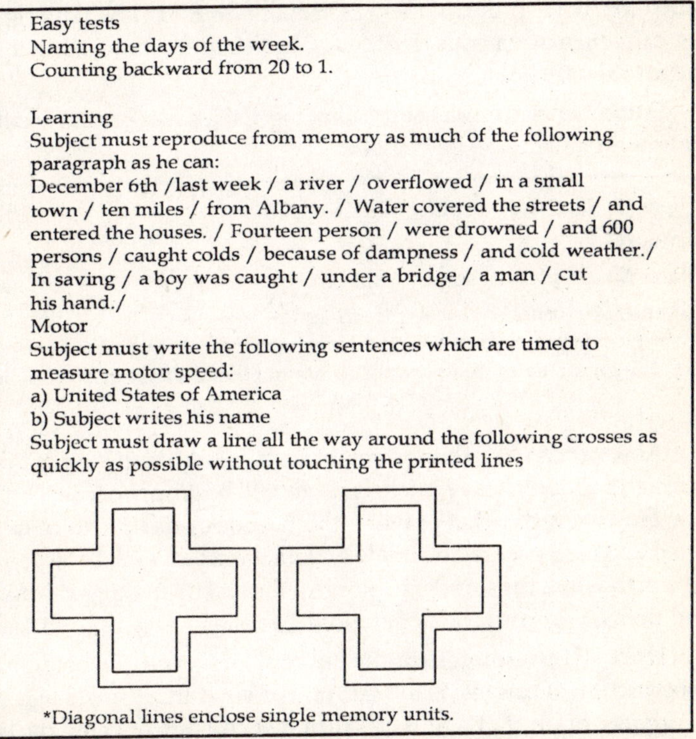

Easy tests
Naming the days of the week.
Counting backward from 20 to 1.

Learning
Subject must reproduce from memory as much of the following paragraph as he can:
December 6th /last week / a river / overflowed / in a small town / ten miles / from Albany. / Water covered the streets / and entered the houses. / Fourteen person / were drowned / and 600 persons / caught colds / because of dampness / and cold weather./ In saving / a boy was caught / under a bridge / a man / cut his hand./

Motor
Subject must write the following sentences which are timed to measure motor speed:
a) United States of America
b) Subject writes his name
Subject must draw a line all the way around the following crosses as quickly as possible without touching the printed lines

*Diagonal lines enclose single memory units.

Fig. 5.4. Examples of Items on the Babcock-Levy Mental Efficiency Test.

In the future the use of newer types of tests may make this approach more fruitful.

Shipley-Hartford. Some brief mention should be made of this test which is also based on the Babcock principle. It has very limited value because of relatively poor standardization and discriminative power and because it re- quires a rather high vocabulary level and superior intelligence to take successfully. Although the data obtained with the test indicate that chronic psychotics usually show losses and early psychotics may not, the authors nevertheless claim to have intended the test for early and mild cases of disturbance.

The Shipley-Hartford consists of two parts, a vocabulary subtest and an abstraction subtest, both of gradually increasing difficulty. An index of impairment is obtained by dividing the abstraction age by the vocabulary age times 100. This index is called the "conceptual quotient." Quotients much below 100 suggest the existence of various degrees of impairment depending upon the actual value obtained.

Subject must complete the following. Each dash (-) calls for either a numberor a letter to be filled in.

Item (3)	AB	BC	CD	D-			
Item (4)	Z	Y	X	W	V	U	-
Item (7)	escape	scape	cape	---			
Item (11)	mist is	wasp as	pint in	tone--			

Fig. 5.5 Examples of Items from The Abstraction Subtest of the Shipley-Hartford Scale.

As it stands now, this test really adds mostly dead weight to the clinician's already heavy satchel and should be dropped from clinical use. However, the idea of using the Babcock principle to obtain a rapid and easily scored estimate of deficit is an excellent one. It may be worth while for someone to revise the test by making it simpler and doing a thorough job of standardization.

Hunt-Minnesota: As in the Babcock, the principle behind the construction of this test is the stability of vocabulary in old age and in organic brain damage. The Hunt test consists of three parts, a vocabulary test, six immediate and delayed-recall tests (the scores of which are compared with vocabulary to obtain an index of impairment), and nine interpolated tests (e.g., information, number counting, an attention test, digit span, and naming months in reverse order). These nine interpolated tests are called the "validity indicators" because patients who are unable to perform them are too uncooperative, disturbed, or deteriorated to produce results which can be properly interpreted.

As in the case of the Shipley-Hartford Scale, this instrument is of very limited value because the author did not spend the time necessary to obtain adequate norms and validity data. Only 33 patients and 41 controls were used in the standardization population. While the test did discriminate reliably between the two groups, the overlap was so large that its use for individual diagnosis is extremely hazardous. The use of the validity indicators represents the real contribution of Hunt's test to the testing of psychotic patients. It is an old psychiatric idea which could have considerable usefulness in diagnostic testing. With revision and the outlay of the necessary labor, the Hunt-Minnesota type of test could be of value in providing a rough estimate of a patient's intellectual deficit.

Concept Tests: As a result of his observations with aphasic patients over a period of many years, Kurt Goldstein has suggested that patients with brain damage show a characteristic loss in abstract ability. He has repeatedly suggested that cerebral lesions always produce this single basic change in functioning. While Goldstein's generalization has been challenged frequently, it has led to some work on the construction of tests designed to measure roughly this abstract loss. The primary purpose of these tests is to pick out patients with organic brain damage.

Goldstein has been a main contributor to the concept tests along with his collaborator Gelb, from whom he borrowed heavily. From the work of these men there has emerged a series of five tests aimed at the identification of patients with brain lesions. These are: the Goldstein-Scheerer Cube Test; the Gelb-Goldstein Color Sorting Test; the Goldstein, Gelb, Weigl, and Scheerer Object Sorting Test; the Weigl-Goldstein-Scheerer Color Form Sorting Test; and the Goldstein-Scheerer Stick Test. In a monograph by Goldstein and Scheerer, the use of these tests is described. In addition another test originally designed in 1934 by Vigotsky and later adapted and used by Hanfmann and Kasanin has been frequently used in the diagnosis of brain damage and schizophrenia.

While these tests have a similar rationale to the deficit tests we have described above, they do not use a reference point against which to compare the individual's abstract functioning. In concept-formation tests it is assumed that the normal subject should be able to solve the problems adequately if he does not have brain damage. The measurement has been an all-or-none affair. The patient's performance is in reality compared with norms in only a qualitative sense. Experience with normal on the tests indicates that most of them can perform at the abstract level to pass them.

Despite their differences, the basic principle behind these tests is very similar to the principle on which pattern and scatter analysis rest. Patients who have brain lesions arc expected to show a dependence on concrete forms of behavior and to fail in the abstract functions. This is essentially saying that some functions are impaired (abstract ones) and others are retained (concrete ones) in patients with brain lesions.

Observations of schizophrenic patients indicate that they, like organics, also fail in the concept tests. The differentiation between an organic patient and a schizophrenic patient cannot therefore be made on the basis of these tests. Other signs must be used. Often the differentiation is made on largely qualitative features like bizarre behavior and lack of the apparent anxiety which characterizes most organic cases. Although they have some value, the concept tests are only suggestive in diagnostic use. Errors of classification are frequent even when the tests are carefully applied. We shall briefly describe each of the concept tests used in the clinic.

The Cube Test was constructed to determine whether the patient can abstract a small design of different colors and copy it in a larger size with four Kohs blocks. The blocks are cubes, colored so that one side is blue, one red, one yellow, one white, one blue and yellow, and one white and red. On the side with the combination, the two colors are divided diagonally across the cube. There are 12 designs to be copied, all of them except one having been taken directly from the Kohs blocks series.

The patient may deal with the Cube Test problem on a concrete or abstract level. He can succeed at an abstract level by making the correct solutions without the aid of a graded series of modified designs which the tester may introduce to help the patient. These modifications for each design, which are not introduced unless the patient fails, involve an enlargement of the model to actual block size, an emphasis on the part relationships by drawing in lines where the separations between the blocks would be, and finally, if these fail, the introduction of a model out of the actual blocks. These aids make the process of abstraction, which the organic patient finds difficult, unnecessary for the solution of the problem. Organic patients have difficulty even when aided by the modified models. There are no objective-scoring criteria to the test. Degrees of impairment may be inferred from the amount of help needed to copy the models or the failure to profit from this help altogether.

The Color Sorting Test requires the subject to sort a set of woolen skeins according to color concepts. The test has four parts. In the first, skeins of different hues and saturations are presented at random to the subject. The testee selects any one and then is asked to pick out of the group all other skeins that go with the one he picked. In part two, three skeins are presented, two of the same hue but differing in saturation and brightness. The third skein differs in hue from the first two, but is of the same saturation or brightness as one of the first pair. The subject is expected to make a selection of which go together on the basis of hue, saturation, or brightness. In the third test the patient is presented with a series of six samples of the same hue, but varying in brightness from lightest to darkest, and a second series of different hues but equivalent brightness. The patient is asked to identify the common quality in each series. In the fourth test, the subject must select all the red skeins, or all the green skeins. In each test the subject is always asked the reason for his particular groupings. Feeble-minded patients or those with abstraction loss, that is, those who perform at the concrete level, fail to sort on the basis of some concept but employ concrete matching procedures (such as matching on the basis of skein length), or make no attempt at solution at all. The intact individual usually deals with each test by selecting groups of skeins on the basis of some concept -- that is, color, saturation, or brightness -- without regard to the other aspects. For example, in the first test the subject may select a red skein and sort with it any skein that contains red, regardless of brightness or saturation. When questioned he will answer that he selected all the red wools. Patients with organic injury often have difficulty with such abstract concepts as color. Here again, no quantitative scoring system has been provided by the authors. The patient's behavior is identified by the examiner as either concrete or abstract.

The Object Sorting Test consists of a group of 30 common objects which are randomly arranged on the table before the subject. It was designed to determine whether a person can sort in accordance with some general concept, shift from one concept to another, and determine the principle of a grouping that is demonstrated by the experimenter.

First the subject is told to pick out any object from the 30. Then he must select all the other objects that he believes should be grouped with the one he picked out. After this has been done, the experimenter selects some of the objects one at a time, asking the subject to add others that belong to the one picked out. Then the subject is asked to put all the objects into groups of his own choosing. When the subject has made his own groupings, he is urged to find still other kinds of groupings. Finally the examiner himself makes a number of groupings and asks the subject to name the concept (class) by which the groupings have been made. In each aspect of the test the subject is always asked to explain his actions to help determine whether he has proceeded on an abstract or concrete basis.

The sorting test may be administered in a number of ways since no standards of administration and scoring are given by the authors. The sorting task is apparently simple for normal individuals and even children of 8 or 9 years of age. Mentally deficient subjects, schizophrenics, and brain-injured patients often fail to sort according to abstract concepts.

Rapaport and his coworkers have worked out a somewhat more quantitative technique of scoring the test to determine for any subject the adequacy of the sorting, the conceptual level of the verbalizations, and the concept span, that is, the inclusiveness of the grouping in terms of looseness or narrowness. For example, if the subject selects objects to go together which do not readily belong or which make the concept too wide, the subject is displaying a loose span. If, on the other hand, the concept includes too little, it is described as narrow. With this type of approach, the test has been used in the clinic with a great variety of types of patients as a means of identifying clinical syndromes. Schafer has described the use of the test in this fashion in a clear and useful way and has provided abundant illustrative case material.

The Color Form Sorting Test follows the same principles as we have seen in Goldstein's other diagnostic devices. It consists of a dozen blocks of three shapes (triangle, square, and circle) and four colors (red, yellow, blue, and green, with the reverse sides white). The subject must first arrange them into groups. He may do this according to color or shape, or may put them into piles to form some irrelevant groupings on the basis of structure (concrete behavior). When he is asked to group them in terms of a different principle, the concept-damaged individual may show failure to shift from one concept to another, even if he has correctly sorted them in the first attempt by either color or form. Moreover, in his verbalizations, he may be unable to identify the basis of his action. Evaluation of this test is also qualitative.

The Stick Test requires the patient to copy printed figures with a set of plastic sticks and then do the same task from memory after a brief exposure to them. Thirty-four figures are presented in a rough scale of difficulty in terms of the number of sticks involved and the complexity of the model. As with the other tests, the patient must explain his action.

The brain-injured subject is likely to identify the stimulus figures in terms of some concrete everyday objects and in severe impairment even distort it in copying so that it is more like the concrete object perceived. For example, presented with a figure like this A, he may describe it spatially as two diagonal lines meeting at the top, or he may call it a roof, which he then proceeds to make with the actual sticks. The latter case represents a tendency to perform at the concrete level. The examiner must evaluate the extent of the concreteness without the benefit of norms or scoring devices.

Prominent among the instruments which have been used to study concept formation and impairment in abstract behavior has been the HanfmannKasanin Test, originally improvised by Vigotsky in 1934, to study schizophrenic thinking. The idea is quite similar to the color-form test. However, it suffers clinically from being so difficult that only people of the highest intelligence level are able to perform it adequately. The test consists of 22 forms in 5 different colors, 6 shapes, 2 heights, and 2 widths. The subject's problem is to sort these forms into four categories according to the principle of volume. The four categories, each labeled with a nonsense syllable, are: tall-wide, flat-wide, tall-narrow, and flat-narrow. The entire set with the nonsense syllables hidden on the reverse side of each block, is put before the subject in a random fashion. The experimenter selects one of the blocks and instructs the subject to pick out all the others that go with it. If the subject sorts according to color, shape, height, or width, he will find more or less than four categories. With each error in sorting he is corrected by turning the blocks up and revealing the nonsense syllables one by one until the subject correctly classifies them all. He must then state the principle of the sorting.

Three levels of performance on the test may be differentiated, depending upon its concreteness. The approach, the amount of help necessary, the successful solution, and the verbalization of the principle at the end determine the evaluation of the subject's performance. As we have seen with other tests of this kind, the technique is primarily a qualitative one, although the task has been submitted to quantitative scoring and simplification. Some clinicians have used the test to obtain observations of the manner in which a patient approaches difficult problems. Such characteristics as persistence, reaction to frustration, and flexibility and rigidity have been observed.

Recently, Zaslow devised a test of sorting behavior which consists of a series of geometric figures ranging in a quantitative scale from a triangle to a circle with fine graduations in between each figure. The subject is presented with the series of figures in one row and must say where the triangle ends and the circle begins. In addition to qualitative behavior in response to this problem, Zaslow points out that a quantitative score of sorting looseness or rigidity may be obtained from this test by counting the number of figures left in the middle grouping. The test may prove useful for some purposes, although too little work has been done with it to allow a present evaluation.

The authors of this series of concept tests which we have described have never made any adequate attempts to standardize their instruments and rarely concerned themselves with the problems of scoring except in a qualitative sense. In cases of severe abstract loss they appear to have some value. The theoretical basis of the method has been open to some question, and the discriminative power of the instruments leaves much to be desired. The concept tests have been criticized mostly for the absence of norms and the lack of reliable, quantitative scales with which to evaluate the performance of individuals. There is no doubt that there are huge individual differences on the part of testees in their manner of approaching the concept tests and their success in dealing with them. These differences appear to be related in some cases to intelligence, in others to the type of disturbance and personality organization. The general problem is a potentially fruitful one. It is a special case in the study of the relationships between the intellectual processes and personality.

Critique of the Measurement of Deficit: In this section we shall try to deal with the various assumptions and technical difficulties involved in the current approaches to the measurement of intellectual deficit. Our emphasis shall be placed on generalized technique and theory rather than on particular instruments.

Psychological measurements, particularly as they apply to cognitive functions, may be analyzed in four main ways: (1) Inter individual and inter group analysis on any single function, that is, John has a higher IQ than Jim, or schizophrenics do more poorly than normal. (2) Intra individual analysis -- John is better at the verbal aspects of intellectual performance than he is on the perceptual-motor side. (3) Interindividual and intergroup comparisons of qualitative features in performance such as reaction time, etc. -- John approaches the task confidently while Jim expresses strong anxiety about the outcome. (4) The response variations of a person within each subscale of a test. This type of analysis is analogous to approach 2 above, in which the absolute level of total performance is considered less important than the variability within the individual and within different instances of performance on the same function. As an example of this latter case we might cite Lazarus, Eriksen and Fonda who have noted that a patient who is threatened by aggressive impulses may show different perceptual accuracy for aggressive stimuli than he does for neutral stimuli even though both perceptual tasks are comparable in difficulty. In other words, the function of perceptual ability shows systematic variation within the individual, depending upon the emotional implications of the stimuli to be perceived. Jastak points out that ignoring such response variation within individuals means throwing away some of the most important data from which an analysis of the personality and the functioning of the individual could be derived.

Some of the assumptions and technical problems which arise in the measurement of intellectual deficit apply to all four of the approaches described, while others are specific to particular ones. Approaches 1 and 3 are more similar in that they are both interindividual. Approaches 2 and 4 have a great deal in common, since they both require examination of intraindividual patterns. The latter two are particularly useful to the clinician, since they are so closely bound up with the problems of individual diagnosis. We shall organize our critical discussion of the measurement of deficit and the clinical use of diagnostic patterns around the following considerations: the functions measured, reference points, standardization, diagnostic classification, and reliability.

Functions Measured: We discussed some of the confusions and disagreements which have arisen concerning the nature of intellectual behavior. We also dealt with the question of what our various tests actually measure. It is not nearly enough to be able to say that schizophrenics tend to fail on tests which involve the task of finding similarities. In order that some light may be thrown on the intellectual process in disturbed patients by this observation, it is important to know something about how the task of finding similarities is related to other kinds of intellectual measures. In other words, the functions which we measure must themselves be fully understood in order to make this finding theoretically meaningful. Some psychologists have attempted to make a start in this direction through intercorrelational or factor-analysis techniques. Yet it does at least offer something more solid than the intuitive approach on which clinical psychologists have entirely depended for many years.

The theoretical difficulties encountered by our lack of complete knowledge concerning the nature of our various tests afford a major stumbling block in the diagnostic use of patterns of performance within individuals. The tests we have available today have been constructed by the use of a priori, intuitive classifications of the intellectual functions and on the basis of empirical prediction. The Binet, for example, is most inappropriate for pattern or scatter analysis. The test is a hodgepodge of different types of subtests scattered almost at random. Major disagreement may be found as to which subtests should be grouped together in analyzing the types of tasks failed by various types of patients.

Most important of all, the subtests of the Binet are quite homogeneous. McNemar in factor analyzing the test found all the items to be heavily saturated with one general factor. To the extent that each subtest is measuring a high percentage of the same thing, pattern analysis is inefficient. Subtest heterogeneity is needed before a study of intertest patterns (and therefore the measurement of differential functioning within the same individual) is meaningful. The paradox is that to establish that actual deficit or impairment of function is present requires that the premorbid reference point (e.g., vocabulary) be highly correlated with the other subtests under conditions of normal mental functioning. However, in order to make use of patterns to study differential functioning, it is most efficient to employ uncorrelated subtests; the pattern must then be related to other personality variables. To require both functions of the same test works against the efficiency of each.

Probably none of our present-day tests approach the ideal of subtest heterogeneity. Even the subtcsts of the Wechsler-Bellevue are highly intercorrelated. The Wechsler comes closer to the type of test which could be used for pattern analysis. Although the ideal of pure tests will probably not be achieved, substantial improvements are likely to be made in the direction of more clearly specifying the functions that are being measured and obtaining greater independence among the subtest measures.

Reference Points: As we have elaborated earlier, the study of intertest patterns and scatter developed out of the observation that some subtests appear to hold up and others to show losses in the performance of patients with various mental diseases. Reference points like vocabulary and information from which the scatter or index of efficiency is obtained have their own very severe limitations. Although no one would maintain that vocabulary is not reasonably resistant to impairment, as a good estimate of premorbid capacity it is somewhat questionable. Its use depends, for one thing, upon the definition of intelligence. There is, of course, no real justification in saying that a man with a poor verbal level and a very high performance level has low intelligence. The vogue of using verbal ability as an index of intelligence has serious weaknesses. A person with low verbal and high performance ability might be classified, in our present tests of deficit, as unimpaired if vocabulary were used as a reference point for scatter whatever his state of mental health may be. Even if he had suffered an intellectual loss, this might be obscured because of the initial discrepancy between vocabulary and other functions. This illustrates the need for a high relationship between the reference point and the critical measures of deficit. With our present procedures of using vocabulary as the reference point, we might often be misled in our diagnoses.

Reference points other than vocabulary have been used in scatter and pattern analysis. As we have noted before, the use of the mean of all the subtests or separate means for the verbal and performance subtests as reference points from which to determine impairment has been popular with some clinical psychologists. The main problem here is that this mean is influenced by the deficit, since it is made up of some of the tests which show the extreme deviations. The use of any type of mean reference point is bound to attenuate the deviation because it is affected by the impairment itself.

The various indexes that have been suggested, such as Rabin's schizophrenic index and Wechsler 's hold-don't hold technique, are probably on the right track, particularly if they are modified to be ratios instead of difference measures. They need not suffer from the limited definition of premorbid intelligence that is implied in the vocabulary measure, and at the same time they provide a rational approach to the estimate of premorbid capacity. The problem appears to be one of deciding which measures should be used. These must be functions that really hold up during illness and correlate well with the tests used to indicate intellectual loss. Rabin's and Wechsler's attempts were intuitive and partly empirical guesses about what kinds of clusters to use in the analysis. Babcock and Levy's division into learning, memory, and psychomotor tests was still another guess. The approaches of all three are quite similar and have some validity. But the validity is still too low to provide satisfactory clinical prediction.

Jastak and other shave suggested that the selection of clusters can be made more effective by factor-analysis procedures which will allow us to group subtests on the basis of their observed intercorrelations.

Birren has recently presented evidence supporting in part some of the clinical hunches about the diagnostic groupings of the subtests of the Wechsler-Bellevue. In a factor analysis of the test using elderly people, he found that subtests containing a verbal factor like vocabulary and information declined with age less than those which had high factor loadings on visual factors (block design, object assembly, etc.). The reader will recognize that this is, indeed, roughly the kind of grouping which has been suggested by a number of clinicians interested in the diagnosis of intellectual deficit.

The authors tend to agree that more attention must be paid to these intercorrelations. Whether factor analysis is used or not, selection of subtests and clusters of subtests for the purpose of pattern analysis must depend upon the interrelationships found among our various measures. The technique of intercorrelational analysis is not a method of discovery but really a check on the efficiency of our test batteries. It cannot tell us which types of functions we would like to call intelligence, but it can help us decide whether two particular tests measure similar things or whether they are reasonably independent.

Standardization: Whether intraindividual or interindividual approaches are used, norms must always be provided as a standard against which to interpret a particular score or pattern. It does not help us to know that a patient does better in performance tasks than in verbal tasks unless we know what to expect from other people with various personality characteristics.

One of the great deficiencies of the measurement of deficit has been the lack of adequate standardization of the patterns and deficit scores. Much of this is the result of difficulties in getting large and homogeneous populations to work with. The average clinical psychologist is limited by the particular clinic or hospital population with which he works, as well as by his own lack of time to do the enormous labor involved in the standardization of these kinds of measures. In many instances the lack of norms seems to be a matter of the failure to appreciate the need.

To further complicate matters, there are tremendous problems concerning the classification of patients according to mental diseases. The classifications are extremely variable from hospital to hospital and even within the same institution. Moreover, the same

Table 5.1. The Test-retest Reliability of the Wechsler-bellevue Reported in the Literature and in the Present Study

Author	Gibby†	Rabin	Hamister	Rabin	Hamister	Rabin	Canter	Aborn and Derner	Aborn and Derner	Canter	Aborn, Derner and Canter
	(5)	(13)	(7)	(14)	(7)	(13)	(1)				
Population	Psychoneurotics	Schizophrenics	Schizoiphrenics	Miscellaneous diagno-	Miscellaneous diagno- schizophrenics	Miscellaneous diagnoses non-	Multiple sclerotics	Normals, 1-week retest	Normals, 4-week retest	Normals, 6-month retest	Normals, combined average
N	32	30	34	60	53	30	47	60	60	38	158
					Coefficients of reliability						
Subtests											
Information	.56	.89	.94	.99	.94	.89	.81	.87	.84	.87	.86
Comprehension	.20	.12	.78	.44	.76	.62	.76	.70	.74	.77	.74
Digit span	.65	.62	.63	.77	.59	.75	.73	.67	.70	.64	.67
Arithmetic	.76	.75	.87	.68	.87	.73	.74	.57	.53	.74	.62
Similarities	.71	.38	.84	.62	.86	.79	.93	.65	.76	.70	.71
Vocabulary	.93	....	.90	....	.90	....	.90	.91	.88	.83	.88
Picture arrangement	.49	.54	.78	.60	.73	.73	.86	.68	.59	.66	.64

Picture completion	.87	.32	.68	.89	.71	.80	.73	.80	.85	.82	.83
Block design	.87	.71	.67	65	.71	.70	.82	.88	.84	.78	.84
Object assembly	.53	.31	.62	.67	.66	.79	.74	.73	.62	.73	.69
Digit symbol	.81	.34	.79	.74	.80	.91	.90	.78	.76	.85	.80
Scales											
Verbal IQ	.76	.78	.91	.89	.91	.87	.84	.84	.84	.84	.84
Performance IQ	.82	.52	.80	.76	.83	.94	.90	.88	.83	.87	.86
Full scale IQ	.87	.55	.84	.84	.87	.87	.90	.91	.87	.91	.90

patient will behave quite differently while in different phases of his psychosis. The degree of contact evidenced by one schizophrenic patient may be considerably different from that of another.

All these factors conspire to make the normative problem very difficult to solve. In a large measure they account for much of the confusion and disagreement between the various studies of deficit. If normative studies do not agree concerning the type of pattern shown by the obsessive-compulsive or hysteric patient, for example, then pattern analysis cannot be used fruitfully in diagnostic work.

Diagnostic Classification: Many writers, including the present authors, believe that part of the difficulty in this area lies with the present system of diagnostic classification. The validity of most of the pattern-analysis techniques has been tested on an outworn and unreliable system of classification. While almost everyone seems to agree that we should describe a patient in terms of the dynamics of his problem, that is, a description of the motive systems and ways of dealing with conflict that the patient uses, clinical psychologists are still validating pattern analysis against psychiatric diagnosis as the criterion.

A good example of this approach to the validation of patterns is a study by Levine. Using a group of judges he obtained significant agreement between the psychiatric diagnosis of schizophrenia and the Wechsler-Bellevue subtest pattern. But an examination of the degree of agreement suggests that this diagnostic technique could hardly be practical in a clinical situation. For example, averaging the results of all judges, the agreement was 63.18 per cent. Chance agreement would have been 51.2 per cent. The amount of error in this most simple two-category problem (is the patient schizophrenic or not?) was nearly 37 per cent. It is impossible to tell whether the subtest patterns are inaccurate, the diagnostic labels are incorrect, the judges are inept, or all three. Why should we assume that such diagnostic labels are any more correct, reliable, or meaningful than the very scatter patterns which we derive from the patient's performance? Overdoing this kind of validation procedure seems to us to be attempting to check one doubtful concept against another which is certainly just as questionable. It is high time that clinical psychologists seriously abandon the use of the old diagnostic labels for this purpose. The alternative is, indeed, a most difficult kind of undertaking and a challenge to the modern research clinician.

Reliability: One of the basic reasons for the weakness in the pattern analysis technique is the low reliability of many of the subtests. However good the rationale for this sort of analysis may be, if the error of measurement of each subtest is large, then the entire procedure must have low validity. In other words, we could never be sure we have obtained a reasonably true measure of an individual's level of performance on some psychological function. Often the entire test will show satisfactory reliability, while the individual subtests may not.

One example of this state of affairs is the Wechsler-Bellevue Intelligence Scale, which, as we have noted, is an extremely popular instrument for the use of scatter and pattern analysis. Derner, Aborn and Canter have recently provided a table of reliability coefficients obtained from a large number of studies with the Wechsler test which have used different kinds of subject populations.

The use of normal populations gives generally higher reliabilities than the use of patients, particularly in some of the subtests. Since the test is used largely with patients, the disturbingly low reliabilities in some of the subtests are bound to mean considerable error in interpretation even if the theoretical validity of the technique itself is perfect. Moreover, even in the normal populations, reliability varies tremendously depending upon the subtest involved. The most stable subtests among normal seem to be vocabulary, information, block design, picture completion, and digit symbol. Such subtests as object assembly, digit span, picture arrangement, and arithmetic are extremely unstable and unsuited for this reason for use in individual prediction. Reliabilities below .80 mean that the error of measurement of a test becomes so large that it makes any interpretation of the results hazardous.

What we have said about the Wechsler-Bellevue subtests may be said also of most of the tests used in the measurement of psychometric patterns for diagnosis. In some instances, this vital information is neither supplied by the authors of the test, nor available through others' research. The obvious conclusion is that, if clinical psychologists expect to find dependable techniques of subtest pattern analysis, they must work at devising scales with more reliable subtests.

Summary

We have tried to show some of the reasons why the area of intellectual deficit, particularly as it applies to the problems of individual evaluation, has been so confused. Workers in this field have tended to disagree on the theoretical and often semantic question of what functions they are measuring with their tests. They have used intertest and subtest pattern analysis when the various measures were highly intercorrelated and probably measured much of the same things or when the interrelationships were unknown. In pattern and scatter analysis, questions concerning what sorts of reference points should be used for the determination of impaired performance remain unsettled. In validating diagnostic procedures which make use of measures of capacity, clinical psychologists have also used an unreliable and outmoded system of psychiatric classification as the criterion of the adequacy of the instruments. Finally, even if the bases of the procedures used in diagnostic pattern analysis were entirely sound, the results of the present work would need overhauling because of the unsatisfactory reliabilities of many of the subtests used.

We believe that, despite the difficulties we have discussed, the study of the intellectual functioning of the normal and mentally disturbed individual offers a very bright future for the understanding of the processes involved in illness in general and for the diagnosis of the individual patient himself. While our measures are by no means perfect, their improvement is not only possible, but worth while. It is important that the clinician, who has so much to offer psychology because of his continuous contact and vast experience with the pathological mental states, sharpen his tools of measurement so that they can be more effectively used to study the individual's pattern of intellectual functioning.

6

Psychotherapy in Clinical Psychology

Introduction

Various methods of studying and evaluating the total personality in action have been surveyed. It is obvious to even the casual observer that there are great variations in the ability of individuals to attain a satisfactory living adjustment. On the basis of various criteria, none of which are of themselves satisfactory, a large number of people are referred to as abnormal. They are described as suffering from mental or emotional difficulties or at least as having made abnormal adjustments to life. For diagnostic purposes they are referred to as neurotic or psychotic. The diagnosis, prognosis, and treatment of these conditions are in part psychological problems. The disorders are the result of a long series of processes, hereditary, congenital, and environmental, and complete understanding is dependent upon the examination of all these factors. The difficulties may stem from genetic factors; other causes may have operated in the fetal period; and still others may be found in the interaction between the organism and the environment. A satisfactory understanding of all these conditions, however, requires the participation of the divisions of medical science, psychology, sociology, anthropology, and other disciplines. A complete examination of all these forces is clearly beyond the scope of this book, but some orientation to the problems is essential.

Attempts to view the problems of etiology have been fraught with difficulty that is due primarily to efforts to distinguish between physical and psychological causes. Gandular disturbances, deficiencies in cell nutrients, injuries to nervous tissues, and the introduction of bacteria and toxins may all play roles in personality and behavior disorders. On the other hand, any one who has any acquaintance with habit formation and learning will recognize also that the learning can go wrong and result in personality and behavior disorder. What will be the extent and nature of this disorder will depend in a measure upon the individual's experience with drive and conflict and upon the conditions of his interpersonal relationships. An abundance of evidence has been accumulated to substantiate the fact that structural damage and physical and chemical changes may have marked influence on conscious experience and resulting behavior and conversely that conscious experience may result in physical, chemical, and even body-tissue changes. Such statements may appear to suggest that the difficulty is to be found either in the organism or in its interaction with the environment. No such implication is intended.

Rather it is to be emphasized that physical changes and psychological experiences must be considered for their combined and interrelated influence on the individual. Dunbar and Weiss and English among others have called attention to this point of view. Nevertheless mental disorders are still classified under the major headings of organic and functional disorders, a classification that tends to obscure the important interrelationships. Thus certain disorders involving mental dysfunction may be shown to be due to toxic states, bacterial infections, glandular disturbances, or to neurological damage and are consequently called "organic." In other disorders the function is disturbed, that is, the mental aberrations are present, but they cannot be correlated with organic changes. The abnormalities are believed to be psychogenic in origin, and such disorders are referred to as "functional."

Treatment of illness due to organic causes is a medical problem and will not be discussed here. It is true that clinical psychologists have been interested in such conditions and have participated in the devising, administering, and evaluating of test procedures that attempt to measure the nature and extent of the organic damage as indicated by the loss of psychological functions. They have also worked with such procedures in the interest of differential diagnosis.

Treatment of the functional illnesses is based on psychotherapy; and since such treatment involves real psychological understanding and guidance, the interest of the clinical psychologist has been considerable. The functional disorders are classified under two major divisions, the psychoses and the neuroses. The psychoses include such disorders as schizophrenia (dementia praecox), manic-depressive psychosis, involutional melancholia, and paranoia. The neuroses may be differentiated as anxiety states, anxiety conversion or hysteria, obsessive-compulsive, and phobic states or psychasthenia, etc. Full descriptions of these disorders may be found in textbooks of psychiatry such as Henderson and Gillespie or in textbooks of abnormal psychology, such as Dorcus and Shaffer.

It should be noted, however, that some confusion exists regarding the distinction between the psychoses and the neuroses. Despite some difficulties in differential diagnosis the psychoses are the more serious disturbances, and some differences between the two are readily distinguishable. The psychotics are often poorly oriented for time, place, and person. Although any person may at times be unable to state the exact date, the psychotics may frequently be months or years out of the way. In the same way they may misidentify themselves and be unable to tell where they are. The psychotics sometimes lose contact with reality and evidence great difficulty in separating the products of imagination from those events which take place in reality. Insight into their condition is apt to be poor and in some instances is completely lacking. They are likely also to show serious signs of personality disorganization, as is indicated by delusions and hallucinations.

The neurotics may sometimes be just as seriously disabled, but the disturbances of their psychic life are less severe and the personality does not show the signs of complete disorganization. They are usually well oriented for time, place, and person; and while their insight does not enable them to understand the reasons for their difficulties, they are able to recognize the fact that the difficulties exist. Although their indulgences in fantasy may be extreme, they are able to distinguish fact from fancy. Finally, they do not suffer the extensive disorganization of personality in which delusions and hallucinations are exhibited.

A number of personality and behavior disorders of less serious nature than psychoses or neuroses are of definite interest to clinical psychology. Child delinquencies and maladjustments, marital, scholastic, and occupational difficulties, and many types of failures in interpersonal relationships may require and respond to some form of psychotherapy.

Early organized psychotherapy was centered on the observation, description, and care of severe cases of mental disturbance requiring hospitalization. These cases included, for the most part, the organic and functional psychoses. With the development of deeper understanding of the personality structure, mainly through psychoanalysis, the psychoneurotic became the object of psychiatric study and therapy. The severe chronic neuroses were given more attention, and considerable therapy was practiced outside the hospital. While the recovery and rehabilitation of the chronic neurotics surpass that of the recovery of the psychotics, the time required for recovery and the number of successful efforts leave much to be desired.

More recently there has developed a widespread tendency to extend the psychotherapy to the mild chronic and acute neuroses as well as to the incipient cases of emotional disturbance. Such cases offer the greatest possibility of success, and treatment of them is very important for society. There is also an economy in therapeutic time and effort. The milder cases are greater in number than the severe cases; and since they are not so severely incapacitated, their influence on the social environment is far greater. A large number of emotionally disturbed persons, who may not fall into definite psychiatric classifications, continue to play an active part in social and economic affairs. In the home, in business, in politics, and in social activities, they exert a far-reaching effect which is unhealthy for them and for those in their sphere of influence. Treatment for them is important not only because they are the group most likely to benefit, but also because they affect the personality and mental health of those with whom they are closely associated. The successful handling of an acute neurotic problem may, then, prevent the gradual development of a chronic condition. It may also benefit those in close association with the patient, since they will not be subjected to the stresses of close association with neurotic behavior.

The problems of treatment are extremely complex, and it is therefore not surprising to find many differences of opinion concerning them. The conflicting opinions will show themselves in a great variety of questions that have to do with psychotherapy. The more important questions include the following: What should be the training and background of the therapist? When is therapy indicated? What are the objectives of psychotherapy? What are the explanations of the patient's difficulty? What kinds of therapeutic techniques are most efficacious?

Background and Training of The Psychotherapist

As has already been indicated, the training and background of the psychotherapist is a very controversial topic. No effort will be made here to present all the points of argument, but rather attention will be given to those conditions on which there is general agreement. In doing so, however, some of the points of controversy will inevitably be raised.

It is perhaps obvious that the therapist must know as much as is possible about the causes of the maladjustments that are manifest in the patient. The necessity for a deep understanding of psychological facts and theories is therefore the first essential. Since for the most part the patient is the victim of faulty and incomplete learning, the therapist must have an understanding and appreciation of the various theories of learning. He must be able to evaluate the importance of drive, reinforcement, and extinction. He must be able to appreciate the fact that emotional attitudes may have damaging effects because the patient has no way to label them. The mechanism of repression must be understood as well as the various psychological devices available to the patient for escape from his guilt, fear, anxiety, and conscience.

The therapist must know himself; otherwise the important relationship between himself and the patient is not likely to be satisfactory or successful. Psychoanalytic therapy insists that the therapist first be thoroughly analyzed himself. Such an analysis serves a dual purpose. On the one hand, the analyst learns about his own drives, anxieties, conflicts, transferences, and repressions; and on the other hand, he begins to learn how these are uncovered and dealt with in the therapeutic situation. Other therapeutic systems have not made the same demand for such a complete training analysis, but all insist that the training for therapy include some techniques for better understanding of the self. Some of this may be accomplished by self-study and by the writing of an autobiography which may then be discussed in detail with a trained and competent therapist.

This self-understanding is important, first, in order that the therapist may create an atmosphere of freedom which will enable the patient to communicate his fears and anxieties, reach down to his repressions, and develop important discriminations. The anxieties that have been disabling for the patient are common, in a manner, to all people, including the therapist. Unless the therapist's own anxieties have been allayed and understood, he may show apprehension or anxiety when the patient fearfully communicates his own thoughts and thus he will tend to strengthen rather than weaken the patient's repressive tendencies. Perhaps the greatest dangers associated with the therapist's lack of understanding of himself are apt to develop in the transference. As the therapy proceeds, the patient is likely to transfer some of his emotional attitudes to the person of the therapist. The therapist must be able to recognize the unreasonableness of these responses and to further understand and control his own responses to the patient. He must be in a position to receive and understand the patient's communications and be able to help him make discriminations. His own anxieties, repressions, and unconscious motivations can seriously interfere with the therapy. Even after a thorough analysis or understanding of the self, the therapist must continually be on guard to prevent his own problems from interfering with the progress of his therapeutic endeavors. His own aggressions and fears may make him stiff and unbending, and his own impulses to protect may likewise interfere with therapeutic progress. Therefore, whenever his own behavior in the therapeutic situation deviates from his rational plan, he may find it necessary to examine his unconscious motivations.

In addition to a broad knowledge of psychological theory and an understanding of himself, the therapist is aided by a real understanding of social conditions and their effect on personality development. Most people have a fairly satisfactory knowledge of the social conditions in which they, themselves, have developed but little understanding of the effects of other social or cultural conditions. This lack of understanding does not apply only to markedly different cultures but also to the different levels of social conditions within any particular culture. Lower-, middle-, and upper-class groups live under different social conditions, and their personality development may consequently be expected to be influenced by these conditions. The crossovers that many individuals make, living at one time with those who have developed under the influence of lower-class social conditions and at another time with those who have developed under upper-class social conditions, are the simplest illustration of the social understanding that is necessary for the therapist. Since social-class frustrations may contribute to the psychopathology of the individual, it is important that the therapist understand the social stresses to which the patient has been subjected. Otherwise he may attribute certain conditions in the patient's experience to unconscious forces rather than to social forces in the patient's environment. Behavior that is tolerated in one social group causes guilt and anxiety 295in another. 295The broader the understanding of social and cultural forces, the better is the position of the therapist for the understanding and guidance of his patient.

The therapist must, of course, be a master of the techniques and strategy that are the tools for therapy. These techniques and the strategy involved are, in fact, the subject matter for later chapters and will be only briefly referred to here. The therapist, whatever his special bent, must understand the techniques and values of suggestion, reassurance, catharsis, free association and transference, desensitization, reeducation, interpretation, synthesis, etc., and must know when they can be most effectively used. Such understanding is developed in part from the psychological, cultural, and self studies already referred to and in part from the specific study of all the special techniques. Good ability, however, must wait upon actual experience in carrying out therapeutic work under expert guidance. The therapist must receive special training in psychotherapy. This may be accomplished in a variety of ways. He needs to have the opportunity to discuss the theory and practice of psychotherapy in special seminars. One of the most valuable training devices in any field is that of making available to the trainee the work of a master. Thus the sound recordings of the work of a competent therapist may be made available to the trainee along with the opportunity to discuss the techniques that have been demonstrated and errors into which a novice might fall. He may also have recordings made of his own therapeutic interviews and discuss with his supervisor the errors and successes that are evident in his early practice. In the examination, discussion, and practice situations, he must learn such important things as when supportive or insight therapy is indicated, which techniques should be utilized, when restraint is necessary in regard to his own participation, when to intervene, and when to use the great variety of attitudes that constitute the strategy of the therapeutic situation.

The therapist must be able to discriminate between functional and physical causation, or if unable to do so, he must collaborate with someone who may make such discrimination. Since organic changes may result in mental disturbances, the possible organic factors must be understood, or the therapist may make the dangerous error of attempting to apply psychological treatment to organic causes. The ability to make this discrimination is also necessary, since one of the most common and swift recourses of the neurotic patient is to physical symptomatology. These symptoms must be carefully evaluated in every therapeutic situation.

The medically trained therapist may decide to determine for himself whether somatic factors are involved in the patient's complaint. In like manner, when somatic symptoms arise in the course of the psychotherapy, the medical therapist may diagnose them himself. In many instances, however, even the medical therapist does not choose to make all these discriminations himself but prefers to call on medical specialists. Indeed, many psychiatrists prefer to have even the more routine physical examinations done by other medical colleagues. Some psychiatrists make this decision because they believe that the time given to psychotherapy is so extensive as to prevent sufficient continuing experience in the diagnosing and evaluating of somatic illness. Still others believe that better rapport is established with their patients when the medical decisions are made by another physician.

The non medical therapist or clinical psychologist should insist upon a preliminary medical examination. This should be done whether somatic involvement is suspected or not. In the course of the psychotherapy it may be necessary to refer the patient several times to medical specialists for the determination of organic complications. When such referrals are made, it is important that the consultant not become involved in the psychotherapy. In some cases the therapy requires both medical treatment and psychotherapy, in which case the treatment should be carried on by a medical therapist or at least under his supervision.

Psychotherapy as a professional technique belongs primarily to the field of psychiatry, that branch of medical science dealing with the diagnosis, care, and treatment of mental illness. The psychiatrist is required, therefore, to be trained in psychological understanding as well as in medicine. More recently many psychologists with special background and training have become interested in therapy. The distinction between such psychologists and psychiatrists is not always clear-cut. Psychiatry deals with diagnosis, classification, and treatment, whereas abnormal psychology may be considered to be the science that formulates rules and principles applicable to abnormal and unusual forms of behavior. Such distinction of fields might lead us to believe that psychiatrists would be concerned with the treatment and psychologists with the formulation of hypotheses and the submitting of these to experimental tests. In practice both groups engage in both types of work. Investigators in psychology are constantly demonstrating the relationship existing between mental activity and physiological activity and organic conditions. Psychiatrists, as well as general medical researchers, present facts of physical and mental relationships and contribute to the research in abnormal psychology. In the same way the interest of the psychologist in the development of abnormality is carried over into the treatment of abnormal individuals.

Competence in psychotherapy does not come automatically with the attaining of a medical degree or a Ph.D. in psychology. It is acquired only with a special kind of training, some of the elements of which have been briefly described here. Both medical science and psychology have contributed to the development of this training, which is as yet far from complete. Much more study is necessary before we can develop sound understanding of the kind of scientific knowledge on which psychotherapeutic procedures should rest. In any event, it is important for the clinical psychologist who engages in psychotherapy to be cognizant of his limitations and of the necessity for the consultations which these limitations demand.

Objectives of Psychotherapy

The objectives of psychotherapy have been stated in many ways, but an examination of the terms used often shows differences of psychological theory or method rather than differences in objectives. Thus the objectives may be stated in terms of affective, security, or power goals, depending upon which of these factors has been given greater prominence in the psychodynamic theory. Some authorities state the goals in terms of the possible outcome of a particular method or the degree of change that may appear to be possible in a particular person. Actually the objective of psychotherapy is always the same, namely, to secure the soundest degree of mental or psychological health that is possible. This general objective, however, involves a number of specifics that are obtained in part by enabling the individual to manage his own ego-defense system satisfactorily; in part, by reducing his emotional stresses and making it possible for him to face new experiences objectively; and in part, by helping him to deal with his dynamic drives in ways that are socially acceptable and will result in satisfactory interpersonal relationships.

The ultimate goals include the development of understanding, the release of personal resources, and continuous growth in social adjustment. The neurotic person has developed naïve, rigid defensive habits of dealing with his dynamic needs. He must uncover the meaning and purpose of his symptomatic behavior, develop understanding of his repressions and ego defenses, and find more satisfying ways of dealing with his anxieties. The objective is not to solve a problem or a series of problems but rather to provide for a situation of continuous growth or change so that new problems and recurring problems may be met adequately. The individual must acquire an appreciation of his conscious and unconscious motivations and through corrective emotional experience must develop a sense of security and feelings of personal worth and adequacy. The continuous growth should relieve the patient of his infantilism and enable him to meet anxiety-laden situations with emotional maturity.

The accomplishment of these objectives is not a simple task, and success is dependent upon a number of factors. The adroitness of the therapist, the extent to which the environment is favorable or modifiable, the resources of the patient, and the degree to which the patterns of the illness are modifiable will all enter into the possibility of success.

The goals set for any particular treatment must always depend upon a sound knowledge and understanding of the psychodynamic principles involved. Only on the basis of such understanding can a plan be developed for the treatment. Some things may need to be done immediately, or progress will be impossible; some things must be avoided to prevent therapeutic disaster. Yet the choice cannot be made without genuine understanding. Some of the necessary understandings may be obtainable directly from the patient; others will come through those close to the patient and by examination of the patient's record of living and the conditions under which this record was made. Still others will be obtained through physical and psychological diagnostic tests and examinations. With such knowledge in hand, it is possible to come to some general decision regarding the possible goals and methods to be utilized for obtaining them.

The method of therapy to be used may then be related to the objectives or possible goals. In general, two types of therapy, insight and supportive, may be distinguished. "Insight" or "uncovering" therapy describes those treatments in which there is an effort to bring about a permanent change in the ego by developing the patient's insight into the reasons for his difficulty. The method also promotes emotional growth and understanding and consequently brings about an increasing ability of the ego to achieve satisfactory life adjustments. If the treatment is arranged to give support to the ego, rather than to bring about permanent ego changes, it is called "supportive." While it is possible to deal entirely in terms of either support or insight, this situation seldom occurs and most treatments involve both approaches. The terminology is, however, useful in distinguishing one major effort from another.

While some support is inevitably present in all insight therapy and some insight is obtained in all supportive treatment, the therapy can be best planned when the therapist has decided which of these objectives is to be uppermost. Supportive therapy is used in certain acute cases where it is clear that the ego's functional efficiency is only temporarily impaired. Persons who have been well adjusted most of their lives and who become maladjusted or develop acute neurotic disturbance as a result of extremely difficult environmental circumstances may require only support for the reestablishment of healthy personality attitudes. The long history of satisfactory functioning shows that no permanent change in the ego is needed. The support of the therapeutic situation enables the patient to reduce the intensity of his anxieties and to regain the self-confidence necessary for the adjustments that he must make. In the course of such treatment, the patient will develop some insight and understanding of his acute maladjustment, but the fact that he has been capable of good adaptive behavior will make unnecessary the longer insight or uncovering analysis.

Supportive therapy may also be called for with certain severe chronic cases in which the illness is so long standing, the resources for health so poor, and environmental blocks so great that there is practically no hope of effecting a permanent change. Such people may have to receive some assistance and guidance most of their lives. The guilt, anxiety, and inferiority feelings cannot be traced back to the source, but rather must be assuaged by the permissivity, protection, and reassurance of the therapeutic situation. Thus support is not expected to bring about a synthesis of the personality or provide for satisfactory adjustment that is lasting. It merely tends to strengthen the patient's spontaneous defenses and provide at least temporary and relatively satisfactory adjustment.

Insight or uncovering therapy is, of course, the preferred treatment for most adjustive difficulties. The objective is to increase the integrative faculty of the ego and to rid the patient of his fixed neurotic defenses, thus freeing him for flexible adaptative behavior. This kind of insight cannot be attained by simple intellectual discovery but requires the longer and more painstaking procedure of exposing the patient's ego to various emotional attitudes and situations. The patient must bring to the fore the emotional situations which he has been unable to face, those which he has repressed and around which he has developed his fixed neurotic defenses. The conflicting emotional material must be dealt with first in the therapeutic situation, and the adaptive emotional behavior developed in the therapeutic relationship must be gradually expanded by trial and use in real-life situations. It is an important task of the therapist to determine the degree of insight and support that are necessary and possible in each instance.

Another method used for distinguishing psychotherapies is to refer to them as situational, relationship, or insight therapies. The first of these, as the name implies, is a treatment of the situation. No effort is made to bring about a major change in the person but rather to manipulate the situation so as to relieve the stress. Changes may be made in the patient's occupational or marital status, or he may be uprooted from his environment. For most people the method is not likely to be very satisfactory for a number of reasons. First, major changes in environmental situations and relationships are difficult to accomplish. Second, since a great part of the difficulty probably lies within the individual, the manipulation of the environment is likely to bring only minor relief. In dealing with problems of children, some important situational changes may be necessary, and in very simple adjustment problems of normal people such treatment may be adequate. For the great majority of those who come for treatment much more is necessary, and early situational handling may actually be harmful rather than helpful.

Relationship and insight therapy are concerned primarily with changing the individual. In the former the assumption is made that the change that takes place is due to the relationship that exists between the patient and the therapist. A helpful relationship may be accomplished by catharsis, that is, by getting the patient to discuss his problem and difficulties in a warm and permissive relationship. It may also be accomplished by support through persuasion, suggestion, and reassurance. The individual does not learn much about what goes on within himself but attains better adjustment through satisfactory relationship. Insight therapy, as has already been said, is dependent upon uncovering the difficulties and understanding the factors that are responsible for them. It becomes apparent at once, however, that relationship and insight are not easily distinguishable. Simply knowing the difficulty does not always enable us to deal satisfactorily with it. While it is possible to indicate that one depends more upon relationship in one situation and upon insight in another, both will be involved in most well-planned therapeutic situations.

It is obvious that the objectives of therapy cannot be attended to separately but that they are interrelated in any well-planned therapeutic endeavor. As the therapy proceeds, however, attention will, in part, be focused upon the attempt to penetrate to the root of the disorder and to eliminate the cause. In so doing it may be necessary to attend to some immediate objectives; otherwise the ultimate goal may be impossible. An effort to find the cause, for example, may make it necessary to eliminate symptoms that interfere with progress. However, the symptoms must be recognized only as signposts. The removal of the symptoms does not bring about recovery. Actually there are often contraindications for symptom removal. Substitute symptoms sometimes appear when original symptoms have been removed, and, on occasion, the removal of the symptoms may give the patient sufficient temporary relief to destroy the motivation for continued treatment. In some instances, however, symptoms may be so distressing or incapacitating that it may be necessary to deal with them immediately, or further search for real causes may be impossible. Ultimate objectives may thus occasionally have to wait upon more immediate ones. Other diversions may be necessary in the case of patients who have been inhibited and surrounded with taboos and who need release of vicarious aggressive action. Experimental efforts to improve in social and in occupational experiences may also have to be made.

An unusually instructive account of the principles and goals of insight therapy has been presented by Finesinger. He has not only outlined the steps and the goals but has provided illustrative material that is invaluable for teaching purposes. A number of his contributions deserve special comment. While his ultimate goals are similar to those already discussed, he has outlined a number of intermediate goals under the headings of Adaptation of Physician-Patient Relationship, Production of Material, and Interpretation of Material.

In discussing the physician-patient relationship, he has called particular attention to two aspects that are of fundamental importance. The relationship is seen as providing the support that is necessary and also the tension under which the therapy advances. The relationship is viewed, then, as one that supplies a balance between support and strain. If achievement of the goal is blocked, there may be need for shift in the intermediate goal. In some instances it may be necessary to increase the tension to direct the efforts to the real issue, while in other instances the shift that is required is that of placing more emphasis on support. Intermediate goals regarding the production of material are considered under the following headings: (1) current symptoms or problems, (2) pattern reaction, (3) effect of patterns on current adjustment, (4) meaning and function of patterns, (5) historical development of patterns. Thus the goals follow a certain order beginning with a detailed description of the symptoms. When this has been achieved, the goal is shifted to the attempt to determine whether a certain pattern is unique or a repetition of an organized pattern. When these have been recognized, attention is focused on the effect of these patterns on current behavior. Otherwise the intermediate goals are seen as attempts to understand the reasons why the patient reacts pathologically and the historical development of the patterns. Considerable flexibility is used in dealing with the intermediate goals, but there is no random jumping from goal to goal. It is believed best to pursue a given goal until it is exhausted or gives evidence of becoming unproductive.

Pursuing the intermediate goals the therapist is guided by two principles which Fiseninger calls "the principle of focusing or channeling" and "the principle of minimal activity." The first of these principles is invo.ved with the focusing of the patient's efforts on relevant material. This is accomplished by the display of interest or the withholding of any signs of interest by the therapist which, if adroitly done, results in a channeling of material so as to penetrate the patient's defenses and enable him to bring forward charged material. The second principle is related to the degree of activity on the part of the therapist in the pursuance of the goals. Fiseninger stresses the necessity of minimal activity but calls attention to the fact that this does not mean no activity. The attempt is to keep the activity as low as is consistent with the attainment of the goals. Minimal activity is preferred because it tends to reduce the random participation of the doctor but also because it allows the patient to project his own pattern into the therapeutic relationship and thus provides the basis for better understanding. The minimal activity of the doctor is also seen as useful in enabling the patient to talk more freely in meaningful areas and in reducing the dependency on the doctor. Students of psychotherapeutic goals and methods will find the procedures outlined by Fiseninger provocative and helpful.

Strategy of Therapy

Although the systems of psychoanalysis and distributive analysis and synthesis as well as such devices as suggestion and hypnosis, desensitization and reeducation, and various special therapies are presented as means of accomplishing the goals of psychotherapy, it will be noted that these therapies are not mutually exclusive and that part of each is present in all therapies. Whenever one enters into the therapeutic situation, it is obvious that analysis of the patient is involved. The patient is the object of observation, study, and evaluation; and whether one's technique is that of classical psychoanalysis or not, the treatment cannot continue without some analysis of the psychological factors. In a like manner some synthesizing of the patient's experiences will be a part of all psychotherapeutic situations. The patient is likewise called upon to participate in some new learning and to modify some existing learned patterns of response. Therapy will, therefore, always involve some reeducation. The patient's response to some stimuli must be attenuated; thus desensitization will be attended to. The therapeutic situation itself carries strong suggestive power, and, while the amount of suggestion involved and the conditions under which it is utilized will vary, it will inevitably be present.

It is our intention here to comment generally on what the psychotherapist might do in order to accomplish his objective without regard to the following of the tenets of a particular therapeutic method. The neurotic patient presents himself with a complaint or a series of complaints that are vague and difficult to understand. Neither the patient himself nor those close to him are able to understand the difficulty. People who observe the patient closely are impressed by the fact that he does not make use of his own resources to attain for himself the satisfactions that are his for the taking. Using their own procedures as a point of reference, they feel confident of their ability to advise him of the simple steps necessary for satisfactory adjustment. When these methods cannot be satisfactorily utilized, the behavior is described as stupid. The individual appears to be capable of acting but does not do so. Close observers of neurotic people frequently describe them as "having everything to live for" and are consequently amazed at their inability to enjoy life. The individual appears stupid because he has the resources necessary for attaining mastery in some situations and a strong need for such attainment, but he is unable to enter into competition. Though capable of affection and desirous of obtaining it, he is cold and unresponsive; though physically capable and interested in attaining sex rewards, he is unable to make any satisfactory approach to the area. This stupidity is all the more understandable since it is not descriptive of all the behavior. Although showing average or superior intelligence in some areas, the neurotic appears stupid in others. All the areas of stupidity cannot readily be spotted, and some of the manifest areas may later be recognized as cover-ups for more agonizing areas of difficulty.

The patient also presents a variety of symptoms and complaints. He complains of being unable to sleep, of becoming rapidly fatigued, of irritability, of headaches and nausea, and of being fearful and anxious. If he takes the ordinary risks of life, he is miserable. If he does not take the risks, he is miserable because he does not attain the goals. He is unhappy in all his efforts to approach love, marriage, social experiences, or responsible work situations. If he does not approach these situations, he is disturbed because the satisfactions of such situations are necessary to him. The misery involved is real and must be so recognized. The suffering is due to the fact that the patient is in serious conflict, and the conflict is in part obscured by the symptoms. Strongly driven to attack and to flee, he is unable to act and consequently remains in misery. Much of the conflicting material is not understandable because it is repressed. The competing drives are not labeled so that the patient has no language to describe his conflicting emotions. He is in no position to use his intelligence to solve his problems since he is unable to describe them. Very extensive study of the patient's life may be necessary to unearth the repressions and bring them into focus for study and understanding. Otherwise the patient's difficulties may be understood in terms of faulty or incomplete learning. Again a searching analysis of the development of the personality is necessary in order to become aware of where the learning has gone wrong.

The symptoms and complaints of the patient are the most obvious aspect of his behavior but must be recognized as the signposts and not the sources of the difficulty. They are, however, what the patient brings to the therapeutic situation, what he considers to be the sources of his difficulty, and what he wishes to be rid of. They serve the purpose of reducing the conflict and making it more possible to bear, and their continuance is in part due to this fact. Since the successful symptom reduces the misery, it is reinforced and consequently becomes a learned habit. It does not solve the basic conflict, but it takes the patient some distance from it, and unless the therapist is careful it may also lead him down blind alleys. One of the first things that become evident to the therapist is the fact that the patient's original complaint is frequently some considerable distance from the source of his neurotic difficulty.

The atmosphere or setting of the psychotherapeutic situation must be quite different from that in which the patient has lived and attempted to deal with his neurosis. The dilemma of the patient at the time he presents himself for therapy has been well described by Dollard and Miller.

In the typical patient, his friends and relatives have given up the attempt to help him. Perhaps his physician has also thrown up his hands. The patient himself is becoming hopeless. He has suffered long and tried many cures. All have proved vain. The patient's friends and family have stopped listening to him -- he has complained too long, never able to explain himself. The environment has proved hostile to the expression of his drives, and he fears prudish rejection and gossip if he tries again. Furthermore, he fears criticism of his thoughts if he speaks them out. He feels that people expect him to be unbearably good in thought and act. He has also suffered a series of wounds to his self-esteem. He finds his own thoughts confusing and sometimes menacing. He has lost confidence in his ability to use his mind. He has been humiliated by his many failures to solve real life problems; he has been forced to attempt to adapt in marriage, school, army, or business and has failed. He senses the contempt of others at these failures. No one understands him and he does not understand himself.

The therapeutic environment must be essentially different from the one just described. Since others have given up in their attempts to help him and he himself is without hope, the new environment must provide hope. Since others have stopped listening to him, the new situation must provide the opportunity to talk without interruption. Since he fears criticism, is concerned about his bad thoughts, and has lost his self-esteem, the stage must be set so that he may talk without fear of criticism, express his thoughts without being remonstrated with, and have an opportunity to regain his self esteem. Since he is confused, feels misunderstood, and believes that others hold him in contempt, there must be someone who is not contemptuous of him, who does not consider his statements ridiculous, and who gives promise of understanding him and helping him to understand himself.

The establishment of such an atmosphere is extremely difficult and is open to the possibility of great error. The adroit handling of this difficult situation is what distinguishes the competent psychotherapist from the less successful one. The patient must find in the therapist a person with prestige who presents an attitude of warmth and responsiveness and who listens attentively and sympathetically. The patient is in need of a more satisfactory relationship, and the therapy must begin with the establishment of this relationship and must proceed and progress with the changes in the relationship as indicated in the development of the treatment.

The difficulties surrounding this point may be indicated by considering some of the kinds of relationships that can be and are established. Depending upon the attitude of the therapist, the relationship might be typically physician-patient, parent-child, teacher-pupil, or friend-friend. For accomplishing the purposes of the treatment, any one of such relationships might be seen to have some advantages. The physician-patient relationship is known to us as that in which the physician makes an expert diagnosis and authoritatively prescribes treatment. In our later discussions of suggestive and hypnotic therapy and in treatment of desensitization, it will be noted that this kind of relationship is frequently utilized. The parent-child relationship is one in which there are strong affective ties, the parent taking the role of full responsibility and authority and the child that of dependence. The relationship also suggests relative permanence, at least of the affective ties. In later discussions of psychoanalytic therapy it will be evident that such a relationship is frequently established. The patient looks upon the therapist as father or mother and directs toward him the corresponding emotional responses. The fact that such a role is taken may have something to do with the length of the analysis and with the difficulty of breaking the transference. The pupil- teacher relationship implies that one is to teach and the other to learn and therefore places great stress upon learning and the importance of intellectual processes. In the extreme use of reeducation therapy such a relationship may be established. In still other situations the relationship may be more like the give and take of complete mutuality of two very good friends.

Although no specific therapy sets out to establish a particular relationship for all patients, the therapist sometimes inadvertently does so, and on occasion for specific parts of the therapy a particular relationship is established by design. Actually all these relationships have been experienced by the patient in his life outside of therapy. The patient needs a new kind of relationship, and the therapeutic one at its best does represent something that is different. In fact, it is this difference which makes it difficult to give it a name. We could call it the psychotherapeutic relationship, but choosing a term will not make the situation intelligible. The psychotherapeutic relationship will require further description.

Warmth, responsiveness, sympathetic interest, and understanding are of great importance in establishing rapport and in laying the foundation for a deeper emotional relationship that will be important in the treatment. The patient, who has worn out the interest and sympathy of his friends, finds that the therapist evidences a definite interest in him. In nondirective therapy this is accomplished in part by reflecting back what the patient has said. Questions may also serve as signs of interest and may help to reinforce talking about critical material. The questions are not put forward in nondirective therapy but are prominent in the method of distributive analysis and synthesis and appear less frequently in psychoanalysis.

The atmosphere of the therapeutic relationship is further characterized by a high degree of permissiveness. The patient must learn that all kinds of attitudes may be expressed. The therapist's acceptance of his statements, his calm manner, and the lack of moralistic judgment make this possible. The patient must be encouraged to recognize that feelings of aggression, hatred, antagonism, guilt, and shame may be freely expressed and that they may be directed toward anyone including close members of the family or the therapist himself. These feelings will be expressed once the patient realizes that the ordinary attitudes of social disapproval are not forthcoming. In many instances this may be accomplished by saying nothing but showing no signs of disapproval or shock. While therapists may show great variability in the degree of willingness to answer the patient's questions, it is our opinion that in most instances a calm and objective answer is most desirable. The calmness and reasonableness of the therapist not only reduce anxiety but tend to be imitated by the patient. The permissiveness of the therapeutic situation then reduces the fear and anxieties that keep repressed material from coming to the surface. The permissiveness, however, should relate primarily to the expression of ideas, feelings, and emotions and not to overt behavior.

This is particularly important in treating children by play and release therapy. While an unusual amount of freedom must be allowed the child, regard for the rights of others must be observed, and attention must be given to the kind of social adjustments that eventually must be made.

Reassurance is necessary in all therapeutic situations. It can be a most valuable agent for fear and anxiety reduction. Great care must be taken, however, that the reassurance is not the simple "Pollyanna" type of assuring the patient that everything will be all right or of promising rewards that are not attainable. Such reassurance has already been given by friends and relatives; and when used as a simple supportive device for making the patient feel better, it does nothing but teach him to come for more reassurance or to recognize that your promises are empty. The reassurance must be used to reduce fear so that new thoughts may come to the surface and new acts be tried.

Some suggestion will inevitably be a part of all therapeutic situations. The situation itself, no matter how arranged, carries with it some suggestion. The prestige of the therapist and the confidence that he provides are in part dependent upon implied suggestion. The unobtrusive direction of attention to improvement accomplished but not yet recognized by the patient is frequently helpful. In some situations where the therapy is mainly supportive, suggestive therapy may be used, and on occasion necessary symptom removal may be accomplished in this way. In insight therapy suggestion never plays an important role. In most instances it is important not to remove symptoms since this may provide just enough relief to interrupt the main purpose of the treatment. The use of suggestion and hypnosis for the recovery of amnesic material and for the promotion of a certain kind of catharsis will be discussed in the chapter on psychotherapeutic devices.

The therapeutic situation must revolve about and be dependent upon what the patient has to say. The success of the treatment depends upon understanding the patient, and understanding cannot be accomplished unless the patient talks. The technique of getting the patient to talk and to continue to talk must be the real core of the treatment. It will be remembered that Freud depended first upon a mental purging or catharsis which he later gave up for free association. Great differences exist between the systems of therapy as well as between individual therapists using any one system in the handling of the patient's verbalizations.

In psychoanalysis great emphasis is placed upon free association. The patient is required to say immediately everything that comes to his mind. He must not reject any thought no matter how trivial, embarrassing, or obscene. He is required not to attempt to present material that follows a logical sequence but to say whatever comes to his mind and to try hardest to say that which is most difficult. This obligation is described as the "patient's work" and is applied against the force of neurotic fear. Actually these associations are frequently not free and easy. The patient develops anxiety about some of the associations. He blocks, dodges, suppresses, and becomes mute.

The therapist must provide rewards for talking so that the patient may be kept at his task. Fortunately the permissiveness of the therapeutic situation provides one immediate reward. Being allowed a good turn to talk may be itself a novelty. The therapist is not shocked by what the patient says and does not criticize him. Thus even though fears are aroused in free communication, they may be gradually extinguished, since there is no punishment for them. The therapist must early indicate that the patient will not be judged or punished for his verbalizations, nor will the information be passed on to others. In other situations in which the patient has talked, he has been interrupted, criticized, and condemned. In the new situation this is not so. The patient is encouraged to continue without interruption, criticism, judgment, or condemnation. The patient will now find it possible to talk in the presence of anxiety. He may try out the therapist by saying things about which he is fearful in expectancy of some form of the usual punishment. When such punishment is not forthcoming, his fears about such verbalizations are gradually extinguished. Each bit of material verbalized provides cues for further verbalizations, and using these cues the patient moves step by step to the recovery of latent or repressed material. As the fear and anxieties are reduced, more and more anxiety-laden repressed material comes to the fore. The patient must, however, gradually learn to distinguish between freedom of speech and freedom of thought. There may always be some barriers against freedom of speaking. Speech may have to be guarded in the presence of enemies, before strangers, or before young people. No such barriers are necessary in thinking. It is possible to think freely and to anticipate possible rewards and punishments for action. In this way one may develop the maximum freedom to act adaptively.

The degree to which the therapist participates in this talking period varies considerably both with regard to the type of therapy used and with regard to the stage to which the therapy has progressed. In psychoanalysis, at least in the early stages of the treatment, the patient is seldom interrupted. Later on when more advanced interpretations are being arrived at the therapist may greatly increase his verbal participation. In nondirective therapy the therapist's verbalizations are minimal and are restricted to a particular kind of response throughout the treatment. In distributive analysis and synthesis, the question-answer type of interview is followed, and the verbal participation of the therapist is consequently increased. In supportive therapy the therapist is more active than in insight therapy.

In all instances where real insight therapy is attempted, effort must be directed toward a genuine understanding of the development of the personality. Since there is much that is not known to the patient himself, some special means must be designed to gain for the patient this real understanding. In addition to catharsis and free association, other techniques must be utilized. The patient must uncover repressed material, examine his attitudes from a variety of points of view, learn important discriminations, and finally synthesize his learning so as to develop an understanding that will enable him to meet life satisfactorily. The accomplishment of this goal implies much more activity on the part of the therapist than has thus far been indicated. By catharsis, free association, or even through probing questions, the patient may reach repressed material. He will, however, frequently require help in identifying distortions of his mental life, in developing discriminations, and in correctly labeling emotional responses. The therapist will play a more or less active role in helping him to accomplish these ends. The trained therapist will be able to recognize that certain parts of the story do not make sense, that some important points have been omitted or evaded, and in many instances he will be able tentatively to supply these missing links. In developing this theoretical understanding, the therapist will be guided by a variety of occurrences. At times the patient will be unable to proceed with his associations. When such blocking takes place, the therapist may offer tentative interpretations. Similarly, the therapist may intervene if the patient leaves unmentioned some whole area of behavior common to all people. Slips of the tongue and other errors may also point the way to repressed material; and while in most instances the patient will be expected to develop his understanding through free association, in many therapeutic situations the therapist gives rather active help to the development of interpretation.

Since the therapeutic situation is in part a learning process, much of the therapy will be concerned with teaching new discriminations. Depending on the system and on the individual therapist will be the degree of activity utilized by the therapist in teaching these discriminations. As the patient relates his story, attention must be directed to relevant points. The patient's present inhibitions may be contrasted with the lack of punishment in his present environment. Attention may be directed to his capacity as compared with his attempt to accomplish, and particular attention is given to the effort to encourage the patient to experiment with a variety of points of view with regard to each fact of experience. The success of the therapy will depend in a great measure upon the adroitness with which the therapist handles this and other critical situations. Interpretations must not be presented too early in the treatment. They should first be presented as tentative hypotheses, subject to change as new facts are learned. They should not be forced upon the patient but presented to him for examination and study.

The patient projects upon the analyst the emotions which he has experienced with regard to other people, especially his parents. In the transference neurosis the whole infantile experience with all its attitudes and taboos is repeated, and in the classical psychoanalytic situation this is the essential feature of the treatment. Whether one uses the psychoanalytic method or not, it is important to recognize that the permissive conditions of therapy result in the direction of strong emotions toward the person of the therapist. These responses are frequently those which have long been inhibited and for which the patient has not satisfactory understanding. Consequently by helping the patient to label these emotions, the therapist makes it possible for the patient to utilize them in his reasoning and future progress.

It is seldom true in therapy that mere analysis results in recovery and reorganization of the personality. Eventually there must be some organizing and pulling together of important findings resulting in a synthesis of the personality. It is probably true that the synthesizing tendency of the human personality enables some patients to make spontaneously some constructive use of the material brought forward in analysis. In most patients, however, the illness prevents the ready functioning of associative healing tendencies and makes it incumbent upon the therapist to guide the patient's synthesis. Therapeutic systems differ in their methods and timing in developing the synthesis. Psychoanalysis allows for a long period of free association and the development of transference before interpretation and direction of discrimination. Distributive analysis and synthesis prefers to direct the patient to a synthesizing review after every analysis of situations or symptoms. This is true whether the synthesizing review seems to be called for after one consultation or after several.

Another point in which there is considerable difference in practice is the degree to which the therapist participates in decisions and control of the patient's life outside the therapeutic hour. Nondirective therapy takes the position that the therapy is most effective when the therapist does not take such responsibilities. Definite limitations are set up and made clearly understood to the patient in the early part of the treatment, but the therapist believes that it is unwise to intervene in the environment in the patient's behalf.

Most psychoanalytic therapists also prefer a minimum of participation in the patient's environmental control. When the patients who are being analyzed are hospitalized, the responsibility for environmental manipulation and decision is placed upon an administrative staff member who is not involved in the therapy.

When treating patients who are not hospitalized, the analyst does put some restrictions on environmental behavior. This is usually done early in the therapy to prevent the possibility of precipitate actions that may have damaging effects. Thus the patient is told not to change his job or his marital status or make other important decisions until a better understanding of his motivations has been attained. These directions are frequently changed later as the patient becomes more able both to make satisfactory decisions and to receive the unobtrusive help of the analyst in so doing.

In distributive analysis and synthesis, the necessity to develop a continuing synthesis may bring the therapist into more active relationship to present environmental adjustments. In frank reeducation therapy the therapeutic sessions may actually be spaced so as to allow the patient to put into practice what he has learned in therapy. In supportive therapy the therapist is more active with regard to the patient's outside life, and in shorter course therapy that is psychoanalytically oriented the analyst will be found taking a more active role in the patient's manipulation of the environment.

In any event, no matter what the therapeutic method, the final test is the ability of the patient to make a satisfactory adjustment to real life. The neurotic, or the person with personality disorder, has given up systematic efforts to use trial-and-error methods to overcome his difficulties and solve his problems. In some cases very little help is needed, and the temporary support provided by the therapist may enable the patient to make new and realistic attempts to settle difficult life problems of adjustment. At the other extreme are the more severe disturbances in which every change in the environment is responded to with neurotic escapes. Between these two extremes we find all degrees of difficulty. In the less severe cases a great part of the therapy may be expected to take place outside the therapeutic hour. In more severe cases the therapeutic sessions must prepare the patient for the meeting of outside experiences, and as the treatment progresses, more and more dependence may be placed upon the valuable effects that result from real-life experiences. The experiences in the therapeutic hour are a preparation for later use, and sooner or later the patient must be led to engage in new experimentation in the meeting of the realities of living. He will finally have to solve his own problems with his family, his superiors, his competitors; and the sooner he may be led to approach these, the better.

While there are great dangers to over activity on the part of the therapist, it is possible that passivity has been overstressed. In the treatment of most patients, the time arrives when the therapist must encourage the patient to participate in those activities which he has avoided in the past. There can be no more powerful therapeutic force than the performance of activities formerly impossible. Each success encourages new trials, decreases fear and anxieties and feelings of inferiority and resentment. The success in the therapeutic hour is in part a rehearsal which must be followed by actual performance. No insight or emotional discharge can be as rewarding as accomplishment in real life. The rule of no important changes in life situations during the treatment is founded on firm ground and must be carefully attended to. If this is not attended to, the patient whose sexual anxieties have been relieved might rush impulsively into promiscuous activities; or the timid person who learns about the necessity of standing up for his own rights might behave impulsively in so aggressive a fashion as to get himself into even greater difficulties. Yet in certain phases of the treatment the patient may be ready and able to take important steps in real life, and he should not be prevented from doing so simply because he is not through with the treatment. Only experience can guide the therapist in making these important decisions. It must be obvious, however, that at some point in the therapy the patient must experiment with the carrying out of his new learning into actual life performance.

Prognosis for Therapy

The selection of the patients who are most likely to benefit from treatment is difficult because of the lack of any completely satisfactory criteria for such decision. The examination of a number of factors including physical condition, age, intelligence, adaptability, environmental situation, length of illness, motivation for treatment, use of symptoms, etc., will be useful in coming to decisions regarding prognosis as well as the therapeutic approach.

The physical condition of the patient may have serious limiting effects upon any psychotherapeutic effort. It is essential in the beginning that the possible role of any organic disturbance be clearly understood after competent medical examination. Even in situations where the organic factors are not directly responsible for the mental difficulties, chronic or crippling somatic conditions may constitute serious handicaps for satisfactory psychotherapy.

The possible modification of the environmental situation in which the patient moves is another important limiting factor. The therapy may result in the development of understanding and modification of behavior, but if the patient must continue to live in an environment that is threatening and frustrating, he may find it difficult to succeed. If there is no way out of an unwholesome relationship with the family or an impossible marriage, if there is no relief from financial difficulties, if he cannot secure satisfactory employment or work relationships, the conditions are less favorable for treatment. It is conditions like these that have led to the statement, "We take in the patient and treat his relatives."

While it is possible to effect some changes in those with whom the patient must live, the treatment of the whole environment is usually an impossible task. The prognosis may be said to be poor, then, when unfavorable environmental conditions that cannot be reversed or extensively modified have important roles in the development of the neurosis. In this connection it should be noted that each person's assets will also be a determining factor. In general the more the patient has to live for, the more favorable the prognosis. Physical health and strength, beauty, intelligence, education, special abilities, as well as social status, wealth, professional position, and good family relationships will in general tend to facilitate the treatment. These must, however, be examined with regard to what the patient believes about them, since it is their personal meaning to the patient that is important. In any case they are all relative to the person's needs and the kind of competition in which he is involved.

The age of the patient also has important implications for the chances of recovery. Classical psychoanalytic therapy finds that patients beyond the late forties do not respond well to treatment. Since the method requires the tracing back of associations, the mass of psychic material to be examined is too extensive. In all therapies the treatment requires change and new learning. Since young people learn or make changes more easily, youth is an advantage. This does not mean that older people cannot be successfully treated, but only that the prognosis is better for the young who are more easily influenced to change. Very young children, however, are greatly influenced by their close environments, particularly the home environment, and consequently treatment of the child and the environment may have to proceed concurrently. This may involve consultations with the parents and in some instances the removal of the child to an environment that is more favorable for satisfactory development.

Intelligence and education must also be considered in evaluating the treatability of the patient. This does not mean that the higher the intelligence quotient and the amount of formal education, the better the prognosis. However, since much of the treatment involves the use of language, a certain minimum ability to use and respond to language is necessary. On the other hand, persons of limited intelligence may be aided in supportive therapy through sympathy and reassurance adroitly utilized.

Of greatest importance, perhaps, is what may be called the patient's adaptability. We need to know a good deal about the individual's typical methods of meeting new situations in life. This requires a rather complete understanding of the life history, particularly with regard to adaptation to new demands. Weaning, first school experiences, puberty, moves to new neighborhoods, early work experience, deaths in the family, sex experience, marriage, etc., are examples of the kind of life situations which may be studied with regard to the individual's adaptability. A study of the way the individual has met these and other crises will make it possible to appraise the integrative capacity of the ego. The person who shows strong adaptive behavior in certain areas at least has given evidence of the possession of something on which to build. The individual whose conflict exists only in one area has a better chance of profiting from the therapy than one whose adaptability has been consistently poor.

It is not enough simply to know that there have been many episodes of poor adaptability; one must also know the conditions under which such difficulties developed. It is necessary to know the severity of the difficulty, the amount of provocation, the number of maladjusted episodes, and the degree of satisfactory adaptation during healthy periods. If, for example, there have been many poor episodes under favorable conditions, the prognosis is not so good as when the situations may be related to unfavorable conditions. The individual with a long history of neurotic episodes that started early in life and have been relatively continuous will have missed much valuable learning and will have formed habitual modes of response that are resistive to change. The fact that the difficulty is continuous suggests that the motives behind it are strong; these are poor prognostic signs. On the other hand, those patients whose difficulties did not appear early and whose episodes have not been continuous have less new learning to do and have not acquired so many bad habits. The likelihood is also that the motivations for neurotic behavior are not so strong, and consequently the patients are in a better position to profit from therapy.

The prognosis is also more favorable if the patient is strongly motivated to do something about his unfortunate condition. It is much better, for example, in the patient who seeks treatment on his own than for one who has to be urged, cajoled, threatened, or finally dragged into the treatment. Similarly, the willingness to make some sacrifices in order to get treatment is a favorable sign of strong motivation.

The effectiveness of the symptoms will influence both the patient's motivation for treatment and the therapist's chances of success. Some symptoms are exceedingly effective in reducing the drives in the neurotic conflict; and although the comfort derived by the patient may be only temporary, his motivation to seek treatment may be weakened. In addition, since such symptoms are strongly reinforced and offer some protection to the patient, they are difficult to deal with in treatment. Added difficulties arise if the patient's symptoms result in his receiving rewards from the environment. Thus the patient with a hysterical paralysis who receives financial rewards for his illness (disability compensation) will have his motivation for treatment reduced and will present a more difficult problem in the treatment situation. Otherwise the symptoms may be expected to increase the motivation for treatment. This is true if the symptoms are very disadvantageous to the patient both with regard to his personal comfort and the problems that they cause in his efforts to adjust to his environment.

Economy of Therapeutic Resources

Important advances have been made in the education of the public to the understanding of mental maladjustments.

Consequently, seeking aid for problems of adjustment is no longer accompanied by the same anxiety and concern that were a part of such action in the past. People are becoming increasingly aware of the fact that emotional disturbances can be given rational treatment. The extension of psychiatric treatment to the mild neuroses and behavior disorders gives also the promise of the increase of our knowledge of the dynamics of psychopathology. Most of the theory of psychopathology has developed from the study of chronically ill people, and there is considerable evidence that the understanding of the dynamics of personality development will be greatly aided by the careful study of those who are mildly ill or those who have been relatively healthy most of their lives.

Because the enlightenment regarding mental and emotional illness has resulted in a great increase in the number of people who seek aid for satisfactory adjustment in life, the number of trained therapists is not sufficient to care for all those who need help. It is necessary, therefore, that a much larger number of competent therapists be trained. However, these therapists must recognize the fact that therapy does not take place only in the therapeutic hour but extends itself throughout the individual's life experiences. The individual must go on living while he is receiving treatment, and what happens to him in these real experiences will have a great effect upon the final outcome. It is this very fact that increases the difficulty of evaluating the efficacy of any particular therapeutic technique. Parents, teachers, ministers, recreation leaders, social workers, employers, relatives, and friends are constantly being utilized as therapists, wittingly or unwittingly. Sometimes the individual takes his problems to these people, and sometimes such people feel a real concern about the individual and try to solve his problems and advise him concerning his behavior. Their counsel may have a far-reaching effect. What is said here should not be construed to mean that anyone may serve satisfactorily as a therapist or to suggest that parents, social workers, ministers, and teachers be set up as therapists. The psychotherapist must be carefully trained both with regard to breadth and specificity. What is implied is that others will be involved in situations that are in a sense therapeutic and that the trained therapist must be concerned about their effectiveness. More specifically it means that the professional therapist must give some of his time to community problems, particularly as they relate themselves to therapeutic and preventive possibilities. The recent attention given by the American Psychiatric Association to "leisure-time activities" is one indication of a recognition of this fact. The help that a professional therapist may give to those who are constantly engaged in situations involving individual and group personality adjustment may prove to be much more valuable than a comparable amount of time spent in dealing with the problems of a single chronically ill person. It is likely also that the therapist engaged in such activity will gain in his own understanding of the dynamics of personality development. The growth of interest in group, play and release, psychodrama and other special therapies is another indication of the recognition of the economy of therapeutic resources so necessary at the present time.

7

Functions of Psychotherapy: General Model

Overview

All psychotherapists work to alleviate human distress and foster more effective functioning. They all build on the same basic elements in the therapeutic relation and in the patient's expectations which, in fair measure, may account for the successes reported by all approaches. But, as we have seen, along with these common elements, psychotherapies differ greatly in their purposes, concepts, and methods. In the present chapter, we will consider one approach, in order to have a better idea of what actually goes on in therapy. For now, we shall put aside concern with how systems of psychotherapy differ in order to know one in depth. Later, we will return to a comparative framework.

The form of psychotherapy we will consider is clearly among the approaches described as "evocative" rather than "directive" by J. D. Frank or "insight oriented" rather than "action-oriented" by London and more in the nature of "reconstructive" than "reeducative" or "supportive" in Wolberg 's terms. This approach depends primarily on verbal communication aiming at increasing self-awareness and with it autonomy and control. Historically and conceptually, this form of therapy derives from psychoanalysis, though tempered importantly by the ideas of client-centered, interpersonal, and cognitive theorists. Though concerned with drives, affects, and the unconscious residues of early experiences, attention is more focused on the more or less conscious wishes, values, and feelings of the person in his current life. Particular interest is given to ego processes and defenses in order to understand the ways the person construes and organizes experience and the concepts he holds of himself, relevant others, and the world in general, in both coping as well as defensive aspects. Adaptive strivings and personality competencies as well as pathological defects concern us. Within the context of psychoanalysis, such an approach has been described as ego-psychological.

The vantage point is that of individual adult psychotherapy with patients who have distressing but not disabling problems. They are neither so disorganized and helpless that they cannot voluntarily seek a helping relationship nor, on the other hand, are their problems so limited that some information, advice, or encouragement can suffice. In diagnostic terms, most would be called neurotic, character disorder, or perhaps borderline patients. Typically, the patients are seen for one, or perhaps two, one-hour sessions a week over a period of not more than forty or fifty weeks. This model is possibly the most commonly used by clinicians, whether psychologists, psychiatrists, or psychiatric social workers and, in its general form, is the model within which most clinicians are trained. Within this broad and somewhat eclectic framework, we can now look more closely at what goes on in individual psychotherapy.

Starting Psychotherapy

Psychotherapy starts with the very first contact between the clinician and the patient, even when the initial interview is intended mainly for the purpose of clinical assessment. The explicit purposes of the initial interview include: (I) establishing the interpersonal relation, i.e., rapport, trust, etc., necessary for this and any further clinical transaction; (2) gaining information about the patient and his problems; (3) giving information about the clinic, its policies, the nature of therapy, and fees, appointments, and the like; and (4) bolstering the patient's resolve to change. The first phase of psychotherapy necessarily involves both parties coming to understand what the other is like and what the conditions of their relation can be. It necessarily covers a number of sessions, which may also include other assessment activities such as psychological testing, interviews with members of the family, etc. But from the beginning, the conditions of psychotherapy exist, namely, a communication of understanding, respect, and a desire to help. During this phase, the therapist learns about the patient, but more important, the patient learns, in general terms at least, what will happen and what is expected of him.

Therapeutic Alliance

For therapy to proceed, the patient must be motivated and willing to exert the needed effort. There are powerful resistances, both overtly in terms of the pain of confronting one's less admirable qualities and covertly since the neurotic adaptation, however uncomfortable, is still familiar and secure and change of any sort is potentially dangerous. The patient falters continuously in his resolve, being torn between hope and fear, between the wish to change and the wish to remain the way he is. Therapy depends on the development of a therapeutic alliance between the therapist and the more rational, health-seeking part of the patient's personality.

The patient can be viewed as if he were two distinct people. One is compulsively driven by neurotic needs, distrustful of preferred help, hopeless and self defeating, and quite unable to see himself and his problems with any detachment. Yet, within the same person is another one, who knows himself to be in pain, driven and irrational, but by that very token he is rational. He has hope and a vision, however vague, of a better future of greater maturity and health. The irrational, sick self may be quite willing to continue that way; the rational, health seeking, self-critical self strives for growth. These facets of the person are in conflict along many fronts, witnessed most immediately by the ambivalent feelings at undertaking therapy.

A therapeutic alliance has to be formed between the therapist and the more rational self. Together they take on the task of uncovering and altering the patient's irrational and sick self, until the whole personality becomes more of one piece, as a rational, integrated, and self-regulating self. This metaphor is of course not meant to suggest a Jeckyl-and-Hyde splitting of the personality into two discrete selves, though phenomenologically the experience of many disturbed people is almost literally of being a battleground between contending forces. Psychological well-being, indeed, is often experienced as being unitary, in harmony with oneself, or, in the current phrase, "together."

Therapy requires the voluntary participation of the patient and a readiness to sacrifice necessary time, effort, and money. It depends on a high level of motivation, both to start and to continue, for there are inevitable trials along the way. At the outset, the patient is sustained by hope and trust, though he may have little notion of what specifically is required of him. Early in the formation of the therapeutic alliance is the necessary task of discovering and accepting what I will call the "fundamental commitment" of psychotherapy; in essence, a willingness to look at oneself fully and honestly. This is the essential part of the patient's contribution to the "therapeutic contract" which defines the mutual obligations of therapist and patient. Let us consider these related matters in turn.

Fundamental Commitment

Psychoanalysts have used the term "the basic rule" to describe the fundamental requirement that the patient allow himself to say anything that enters his mind, without censoring or selecting and without thought as to its possible meaning, the impression it might convey, or whether it is logical or silly. By reducing conscious review, it is hoped that unconscious impulses will emerge in the patient's free associations. The patient who truly will not, or cannot, fulfill the basic rule cannot, in principle at least, be psychoanalyzed. The basic rule requires a peculiarly passive cognitive attitude, akin to the relaxation of controls during sleep, rather than the active processes of normal cognition.

The term "fundamental commitment" shares some meaning with the Freudian "basic rule" though differing importantly in other regards. Essential to both is the notion that the patient is not committed to therapy if he would consciously screen communication. Difficult as it is, the patient must be willing to verbalize thoughts and experiences openly, fully, and non defensively. It is true, of course that there are formidable barriers, both of social convention and unconscious resistances, to such openness and these are the proper focus of therapeutic intervention.

But, from the outset, he must be willing to try to be completely honest in telling what is on his mind, as well as what enters it in the momentary situation. Obviously, conscious deceit is the most patent abuse of the "fundamental commitment."

Beyond a readiness to communicate feelings and experience, the patient must voluntarily examine them. This involves taking the perspective of others, notably and in the first instance the therapist's, and trying to understand what meanings his behavior conveys. The more passive mental attitude, central to the "basic rule" of classical psychoanalysis, is not required. The distinction between a more active and more passive cognitive orientation is important but it can too easily be overstated. Even in classical psychoanalysis active and collaborative efforts are required of the patient, but mainly in order to comprehend and integrate the meanings of his behavior as they emerge through the therapist's interpretations. In the type of therapy being described here, which does not emphasize retrieval of unconscious material, the psychological process is more akin to that required of the analyse and in dealing with the interpretation rather than the production of therapeutic material. The essential quality is the conscious intention to relax defenses against viewing and describing one's inner feelings and experiences. Total honesty is beyond the reach of most of us, before or after therapy, but it is the ideal which defines the fundamental commitment.

Therapeutic Contract

The mutual obligations and understandings between patient and therapist can be described as a "therapeutic contract." In effect, it consists of "If you do this-I'll do that" clauses. Ideally, terms are mutually understood, openly discussed, and freely negotiated by both parties; in fact, there may be unstated expectations, implied conditions and "small-type" clauses. To the extent that understandings differ there will be conflict and ill will in psychotherapy as in any other relation. Where therapy proceeds from unvoiced and contradictory expectations, a "corrupt contract" exists which can be destructive of therapeutic ends. It is important, therefore, that clear agreements which can be lived up to by both parties be reached early in therapy. Usually, however, the contract is formed over several sessions and may be renegotiated and changed later on. It is rarely possible, of course, to state in all details the necessary actions and obligations of patient and therapist. But it is necessary that the basic framework of therapy be openly communicated and understood.

The first and easiest conditions to specify are those concerned with scheduling and fees. An appointment time is set, the fee established, and the frequency of visits decided. The patient agrees to come promptly at these hours, to call sufficiently ahead of time if an appointment must be cancelled, and to pay his bill in some mutually agreeable way. The therapist, on his part, is to be available in the scheduled hours and reachable by phone at other times if there is an emergency. He is to arrange for uninterrupted privacy during the therapy session and protect the patient's confidences later on.

Therapy usually starts with a conditional and open agreement as to the length of the process. Except in some forms of time-limited therapy, the therapist's reply to the patient's understandable concern can only be an honest "I don't know how long it will take," though from experience a possible range can be indicated. Usually, however, arrangements are left tentative in the first session(s), for the essential understanding is that it is a time of assessment and mutual exploration. In effect it is a provisional contract: "Let's get together for a few sessions so that I can get a sense of the problem and see whether I can help and you meanwhile discover whether you really want to work with me." Only after this first phase is the contract for therapy decided.

Other than agreeing to schedule, fee, and the like, which provide the outer structure of the relation the patient's primary obligation is to the fundamental commitment, that without conscious reservation and to the best of his ability he will communicate his feelings and experiences openly and honestly wherever that inquiry might lead. What is actually involved in the process can only be known as time goes by, but the patient has to start with the intent to cooperate in the therapeutic dialogue and with the realization that the process may be painful and time-consuming. This essential facet of the contract is poetically encapsulated in the title of Hannah Green's account of her own treatment, "I never promised you a rose garden."

What does the therapist promise? He agrees to give undivided attention to the patient during the therapy session, to avoid prejudgment, particularly of a moralistic sort, and to use his full knowledge, best judgment, and empathic ability on the patient's behalf. Beyond this, he assures the patient of privacy and confidentiality and that he will not otherwise abuse the patient's trust. The therapist communicates, in general terms at least, his adherence to the ethical principles of his profession.

What does the therapist not promise? Most important, he cannot and does not assure a particular outcome. He will try, he will work toward goals, but he cannot guarantee accomplishment. At best, the outcome can only be conjectured-"Many people find after therapy".

The unsophisticated patient may say outright, "Doctor, after ten sessions will I lose my fear of heights and be able to go mountain-climbing?" The more psychologically minded patient, cognizant of the ways of psychotherapy, phrases it more subtly. But the message is essentially the same can I expect to improve for the effort, time, and money I'm investing?-nor is the question at all unreasonable. Our sympathy, professional pride, and indeed guilt, induce us too frequently to promise more than we can ultimately deliver and the consequences are predictable. The hope and power with which the patient invests us makes it easy indeed to act omnipotent in return. Any suggestion of a sure return on the therapeutic dollar "Ten sessions with me and you can be a champion flagpole sitter!" is not only arrogant and ignores the evidence known to all therapists about the uncertainty of therapeutic outcomes, but obviously contains the seeds of disillusionment.

Honesty, in this as in other facets of the therapeutic contract, is essential. The realities and uncertainties of therapy have to be communicated. At the same time, the therapist must convey his willingness to work and his faith in the patient's potential for growth, if indeed he believes it. If he does not, then he should not take on the patient. Whether rationalized as "it can't do any harm" or justified in any other fashion, the therapist who undertakes psychotherapy under these circumstances is acting cynically and ultimately against the best interests of the patient. He, as the arrogant over-optimist, is operating under a dishonest contract. In between, and difficult to define, is that balance of realistic caution and optimism necessary for a workable and moral therapeutic contract.

Setting Goals

An essential part of the therapeutic contract and of considerable importance in planning the future course of therapy are the goals set up early, even though they may be modified as therapy progresses. Broadly, of course, we strive to relieve distress and foster personal growth. However, these general aims can only be concretely specified in collaboration with the patient. The essential starting point is the patient's view of what should and can be accomplished. He starts with a notion, more or less sharply articulated, of what he wants and expects of therapy, and it is imperative for the psychotherapist to recognize these expectations as early as possible. They may be represented in aims as diverse as "to be happier," "to be more effective in my work," "to get rid of my fear so I can climb mountains," "to get over my hang ups and go to graduate school," "to discover what I really want to do with my life," "to straighten out my marriage," and a thousand similar phrases. Sometimes the purpose is more external and does not reflect any wish on the patient's part to change but rather reflects a response to an external demand, such as "because my boss said he'd fire me if I don't shape up," "because the probation officer insisted," and the like. The stated motives may be mixed, containing different and sometimes contradictory aims; sometimes the manifest reason barely conceals a more vital and urgent motive. And, as commonly happens, the patient may have an undefined sense of distress and inadequacy with no clear vision of a desired future. Whatever the case, however, the therapist's first task is to understand the patient's needs and desires.

Danger lies in the therapist assuming or projecting his own goals and values on the patient. Sooner or later the therapist conveys his view of the patient's problems, the desirable ends toward which they might work together, and his own values as to psychological health. But it is a dangerous deceit for him to assume at the outset that they share values and that the patient comes wanting what he, were he the patient, would want of therapy. Typically, it has been found that patients' goals tend to be more immediate and modest ("to improve my home life and get a better job") than therapists' goals for them ("to become a creative, fully functioning individual"). It is true, of course, that patients can have extravagant expectations ("a new man") compared to those of the therapist ("the same person, but a little less anxious.") Whatever the disparity, the therapist can find himself too readily in the position of the artist who accepts a commission for a painting assuming a mandate for a masterpiece depicting, say, man's repugnance for war, when all the client had in mind was a pleasant piece in mauve, coral, and green to fit the space over the fireplace.

This does not mean, of course, that the therapist or the artist must accept any commission precisely as the client defines it. On the contrary, the therapist is obliged to say which goals he feels are worthy, realistic, and within the scope of his technique. Open discussion is necessary to arrive at mutually agreeable goals, some of which may be more immediate and others more distant, some more feasible and others less likely of attainment.

How do we know what goals are realistic? The most honest answer is that we cannot, for we cannot know the future of a human life. But the clinician can predict, within wide limits, probable trends and the likelihood that one or another therapeutic intervention might alter them. Such predictions proceed from knowledge gained in assessment, whether involving prior interviewing and testing or emerging in the early sessions of therapy. The clinician must integrate information about the particular person with knowledge of general principles of personality functioning and psychotherapy and temper his judgments by reasonable expectations as to probable situational events. As we have seen in earlier chapters, it is far from easy to gain the necessary personalistic understanding, and the resulting predictions are at best risky. Suppose a college senior seeks my help because he wants to go to a professional school, but he is severely anxious and feels profoundly inadequate. At the outset we must discover as much as possible about the nature and possible sources of the anxiety, the student's self-concept and coping resources and his intellectual capacities, interests, and school history. If his history shows marginal grades and perhaps limited abilities, coupled with a tendency to buckle under stress and retreat into emotional despair, it might be quite unrealistic to suppose that he could enter a professional school, with or without therapy, particularly in view of the limited number of applicants now being accepted. Still, therapy could be undertaken in the effort to reduce the painful emotions and strengthen coping mechanisms by discovering some of the conditions and conflicts which might underlie his disturbed feelings and behavior. This, rather than the specific and probably unattainable goal of gaining admittance to a professional school, is a feasible goal.

How one proceeds in therapy derives from the goals sought. If, for example, solving a marital problem is primary, then therapeutic conversations at least initially must focus on the husband-wife relationship. In this case, it might even be advantageous to suggest conjoint sessions rather than individual therapy, if both parties are willing. If a person is in acute despair, then a first task is to reduce the painful affect so that the person can give more attention to other facets of his life. It seems self-evident to say that the destination desired defines the route to be taken. Where therapists differ is in their notions as to how early, on what basis, and how firmly goals and consequently therapeutic strategies are to be defined. Some hold that therapy should start with as open a contract as possible and find its directions as issues arise spontaneously. Such clinicians would minimize the importance of prior assessment information, goal-setting, and planning in therapy, lest the therapist work mechanically to predetermined ends. My view is that the therapist must gain, in collaboration with the patient, a clear though not fixed sense of the end sought and the approach that will be taken. Without such a plan in mind, there is the risk of contradictory expectations and confused wandering. The plan should be open to change as new understandings emerge or conditions change, but at any point the therapist should have a fair sense of where he is at, what he is doing, and why.

Setting Limits

The therapeutic relation is often characterized as permissive, as indeed it is in the sense of allowing the patient a unique opportunity for revealing personal feelings without fear of ridicule, censure, or exposure. However, this does not mean that the patient can do anything he pleases as impulse moves him. There are definite limits. Most obvious are those deriving from the initial terms of the therapeutic contract. The patient is simply not free to arbitrarily break appointments, come or leave at whim, not pay bills, and the like.

Beyond this, the patient must respect the person and property of the therapist. He is free, indeed encouraged, to vent angry feelings, but only verbally. Physical assault on the therapist or damage to office furniture cannot be tolerated. Similarly, feelings of admiration, affection, or love can be openly expressed, but sexual contact is forbidden. The therapeutic alliance differs importantly from the relation between friends, lovers, business partners, a physician and patient, or a priest and parishioner, and its value is reduced as it moves in any of those directions.

Nor is the patient truly free to say anything at all he pleases. Communication is to be directed toward the exploration and understanding of the patient's experiences and feelings. Should he want to chat idly about a recent movie, a baseball game, or such other topic, or indeed remain entirely silent, the patient is reminded that he is avoiding the therapeutic task. Such avoidance is understandable to provide respite from the difficult task of self-confrontation and may reflect involuntary blocks as the patient moves toward painful areas. Inevitably too there may be short periods in any hour that the patient will need and want to take "time out" by commenting on some impersonal topic. But continuing in this way has to be averted.

Now we come to the knottier issue of whether the therapist should limit and control the patient's behavior outside of the therapeutic session. The issue here is not whether he should attempt to influence, which is a proper and inevitable part of therapy, but directly require or prohibit behavior. Thus, a patient may feel that he has gained sufficient certainty to approach his boss for a raise and he explores possible strategies with the therapist; it is entirely appropriate for the therapist to say, "If you feel confident enough, why don't you try it?" But some therapists feel it important to require specific activities or to prohibit others. One notion is that the patient should give his full energy to working on a problem in therapy and hence, as necessary, remove himself from living in it in real life. Thus, therapists have required that husband and wife separate for a period or cease sexual relations. People have been required not to drink, smoke, gamble, and the like as a condition for undertaking therapy for these problems. Whatever reasons are given, I believe that therapists should not limit or determine the patient's outside activities. Clinicians have a clear obligation, of course, to help patients understand the meaning, consequences, and potential dangers of their actions. But prohibition as such, which, if meaningful must be backed by the threat of discontinuing therapy, is rarely if ever justified.

Essential Processes in Psychotherapy

The patient talks about his experiences and feelings, wishes and fantasies, problems he is now facing and memories of the past, anticipated events and plans. Words, silences, and gestures carry his messages, some of which are intended and others unintended. The therapist listens with "evenly hovering attention," trying to comprehend the patient's meanings, noting themes, repetitions, and omissions. He then comments, in ways intended to clarify, extend, or relate (interpret) the patient's communications or simply to stimulate or guide their flow. Thus, there is a continuous communicational transaction between the two. In earlier discussion of assessment interviewing, we considered the need for shared vocabulary, common frames of reference, attention to nonverbal behavior, and a variety of other factors which facilitate communication. All of these are equally relevant in the therapeutic interview, although there is a shift in purpose and correspondingly in form. Perhaps "therapeutic dialogue" is a better term to describe the on-going conversations of psychotherapy, if "interview" suggests the meaning of one person gaining information from the other toward his own ends.

The therapist acts to encourage the flow of communication in different ways. He attempts to reduce inhibition and blocks to free expression by, for example, encouraging relaxation, or calming emotional states-"It is painful to talk about ... but why don't you try to go on?" More explicitly, the therapist can suggest topics for discussion-"You've talked a good deal about your sister, but haven't mentioned your brother. Could you tell me something about him?" Under some circumstances the therapist not only suggests a focus but he may ask the patient to limit his attention to it. "A number of times, you've started to tell me about resentment at ... but each time you got off on another issue. Why don't you tell me everything about ... and don't think about anything else for this hour?" In less direct ways, the therapist can steer the conversation, intentionally or unintentionally. Leaning forward, raising an eyebrow, jotting down a note conveys "tell me more" as well as the words themselves. Experimental studies have shown that speech can be conditioned in interviewlike situations even though the subject may be unaware of the reinforcing cues. Krasner has not inappropriately described the therapist as a social reinforcement machine. In psychotherapy, as in any human encounter, the therapist cannot avoid communicating his own feelings and reactions to the patient's behaviors, despite efforts at neutrality and permissiveness; hence, conditioning of the patient's speech is bound to occur. In principle, however, the therapist should know his own feelings and what he is communicating sufficiently well so that he minimizes inadvertently guiding the patient along lines which more reflect his own needs than the patient's concerns. However, even experienced therapists have heard patients say "I didn't tell you more about ... because I somehow thought it didn't interest you."

Of greatest importance, however, are the comments of the therapist intended to recognize, clarify, or interpret the patient's meanings. This is the major contribution of the therapist and we will consider it further later, but for now we should note that interpretive comments of any form guide the therapeutic conversation toward particular areas, both in content and emphasis. The comment "that made you feel angry, didn't it?" not only underscores the importance of "that" but also encourages the patient to dwell on the subjective experience rather than only the objective description of an event.

Central to the therapeutic dialogue is the communication of such personal meanings. In an earlier paragraph, I used the phrase "convey information" to describe what goes on in a communicative act. The term is not inappropriate, but it is important to note that the information conveyed is of a rather different sort than is usually intended by this phrase by students of human cognition or language. The sentence "The next train leaves at 4 o'clock," conveys an important bit of information for me when I am traveling; the patient's "I arrived at my girl-friend's apartment at 4 o'clock," is relatively trivial unless accompanied by modifiers such as "enthusiastically" or "dreading another confrontation." In general, our concern is less with the "facts" as such but with the meaning they have for the patient in the context of his personal feelings, attitudes, and motives which make them relevant and understandable.

Comprehending such communications requires more than listening to the person with our usual reality-oriented, logical attitudes. Processing the informational bit "4 o'clock" is the same in both illustrations, but it is the essence of the message in the station and a trivial portion in the therapy room. It may well be that the railway employee also has in mind "Oh God, how I hate to say the same stupid things over and over. Can't he read the sign? How I wish I was getting away from all this on the 4 o'clock train!" But unless he forces it on me, all of that message goes unreceived.

As therapist, however, one has to hear beyond the manifest statement and to be able to grasp half-stated, unverbalized, and even unknown meanings. In part, this requires a kind of "empathic listening" which picks up more than is carried by the message content. As any empathic act, it involves sensing in oneself cues aroused by the patient's words and gestures which make it possible to know his experience as he does.

It is difficult here, as in our earlier discussion, to convey fully what is meant by "empathic understanding." In the psychotherapeutic theory of Harry Stack Sullivan the concept of empathy figured prominently. However, at one point he said:

> *I have had a good deal of trouble at times with people of a certain type of educational history; since they cannot refer empathy to vision, hearing, or some other special sense receptor, and since they do not know whether it is transmitted by the ether waves or air waves or whatnot, they find it hard to accept the idea of empathy.... So although empathy may sound mysterious, remember that there is much that sounds mysterious in the universe, only we have gotten used to it; and perhaps you will get used to empathy.*

As we continue to work with a particular patient, we internalize a broader and deeper base for knowing his experience not only from the information he directly conveys, nor even from our inferences based on other material, but directly in terms of our empathic responses. Whatever the mechanism, however, the therapist uses this understanding as a base for interpretative comments which in turn serve as hypotheses for further exploration and ultimately lead, we hope, to increased self-awareness.

Examining Experience

Overall, the therapeutic dialogue centers on the patient's present needs, problems, and life experiences. In the first phase of therapy, much attention is given to the patient's symptoms and problems, to picture fully what is troubling him and why he has sought therapeutic help. In these sessions, the patient describes the circumstances under which his problems are intensified and those which relieve him, when he feels happy and when he feels distressed, in what contexts he feels adequate and when inept; in general, the framework of contingent circumstances which seem to govern his well-being. As time goes on, the emphasis usually broadens from discussion of his focal complaints to wider-ranging considerations of his current life. The patient talks about his family, friends, and colleagues, the interpersonal network within which he lives. The patient describes his work, hobby and recreational interests and his social and political concerns; in general, the full range of matters in which he is involved. Some may be long-standing concerns, others are stimulated by immediate experiences ("Strange, on the way over here I noticed ... and it made me think ..."). The patient will talk about his wishes and expectations of the future as well as his memories of the past as they give context to his present experience ("You know, it wasn't always like this ... I used to ..."). It is literally impossible, of course, to catalog all of the sorts of issues which might be considered even in a brief course of therapy. Many topics are wholly idiosyncratic reflecting the particular patient's unique interests, others bear on the common experiences and concerns of all of us, whether related to sexual love, job ethics, or national security. But whatever the focus, the amount and intensity of attention given it reflect what most concerns the patient in his current life. The examination of such experiences is to understand what meanings they have for the patient and why, in terms of motives, character structures, beliefs, and the like, they occurred. The basic material of the therapeutic dialogue consists of the patient's phenomenal experiences of his present life. In picturing his current experience, the patient reveals his characteristic attitudes and feelings. He also reveals modes of thinking, cognitive styles, characteristic defenses, and other ego processes. Let us examine, for example, the following exchange with a patient in therapy.

Therapist: You look sort of downcast today.

Patient: Yes, I feel miserable. Yesterday was my first day on the new job. Everything was wrong. I couldn't even sleep last night. I may not even go back tomorrow.

Therapist: What happened?

Patient: Everybody ignored me. Nobody seemed to care that I was there; they barely said "hello." I suppose I can do the work OK, and I certainly need the money, but who wants to work in such a place. The vibes were all bad. I don't think there's one person there I could relate to.

Therapist: Can you be sure? You were only there one day.

Patient: Well, I suppose I could give it another try. I didn't really get to meet everyone. But they all looked the same, as if they didn't like me and didn't give a damm about me.

Therapist: You said you didn't sleep last night?

Patient: Yeah, I got to thinking about it, and got to wondering if I had done something wrong. Maybe I gave them the impression that I thought they were a bunch of clods. Anyway, I kept thinking about it, feeling miserable, thinking that maybe I had acted pretty snotty. Aw, the hell with it, I'm not going back....

Even in this brief exchange, we can develop a number of reasonable hypotheses about the person's needs, cognitive style, emotional responsibility, and defenses. The patient greatly wants to feel warmly accepted, even in a work situation which might serve other needs and even before there is a reasonable basis for relationships to be formed. He is quick to sense rejection, though also realizing that he may provoke it. Intellectually, he is quick to over generalize and, emotionally, to overreact. As defense, he retreats from a potentially threatening situation, but not before he has dwelt on it and allowed it to make him miserable. In the course of therapy each of these themes would be explored, not once but likely several times, the therapist encouraging the patient to examine and view himself from different perspectives by offering interpretative hypotheses. In the present episode, attention was called, and quietly at that, only to the tendency to overgeneralize.

Suppose, one might ask the patient actually was snubbed by his new co-workers; suppose, for example, he was the first long-haired student in an office of conservative crewcuts. This fact would, of course, temper our understanding of the event, though it still seems true that he overreacted and did not allow the possibility that a warmer and more pleasant relation could evolve. From the isolated episode, we simply do not know whether there were situational provocations or whether the patient was seriously misconstruing an innocent situation. In general, characteristic needs, defenses, and other personality qualities only become clear as we explore with the patient a broad range of his experiences. Overall, however, we are concerned with the patient's understanding and feelings and only secondarily with "what actually occurred." If by contrast we were to look at the same situation with the eyes of an organizational psychologist, we might note that the patient's office tends to be a closed club which receives newcomers most reluctantly, and this has implications for office morale and productivity; however, as the individual's therapist, our concern is with his over sensitivity and, as seems evident in the particular case, maladaptive way of dealing with new social experiences.

Exploring The Past

In the particular case we have been discussing, it is obviously relevant to know that over years the patient has acted in much the same way on many analogous occasions, or perhaps that, until some particular point, he was less consumed with social acceptance or rejection, readier to absorb social rebuff or better able to stay with and work through potentially awkward relationships. Reviewing the past gives context to understanding the patient's current life and problems. In this sense, historical exploration is a necessary part of the therapeutic process, even though concern centers on the patient's contemporary state.

Kurt Lewin took an essentially ahistorical view, declaring that what was relevant of the past still exists in the present. Hence, full analysis of the current "life space" of the person can provide ample base for understanding contemporary behavior. At the other extreme, faith in historical determinism was best defended by classical psychoanalysis. Personality was believed to be formed in the emotional transactions of the earliest years; by the age of five or six, and certainly by adolescence, the personality has its adult qualities. Consequently, profound changes in character organization and genuine alteration of neurotic behaviors require delving into the distant, now unconscious, past to locate the root causes of present symptoms and behavior.

From our present perspective, both positions are too extreme. We can never know the current life space with such microscopic accuracy that knowledge is not extended by discovering historical antecedents. It is true that much that happened in the past is irrelevant; past events as such, in the life of a person or a nation, are not a sufficient base for predicting future history. Moreover, personality is a constantly evolving process, always capable of change, although early emotional experiences are surely of great importance. Indeed, if psychotherapy is effective it is direct evidence of the possibility of new learning in a contemporary relation with another person.

Psychotherapy does not depend, as I have already noted, simply on the recovery of repressed memories. Indeed, much of what is conceived as repressed and unconscious may well be more properly viewed as material which belongs to another, now irrelevant, context and hence cannot be retrieved. Thus, if you ask me to name the streets, landmarks, and events I experienced in a town in which I lived twenty years ago, I may well have very limited recall. But should I visit the place, suddenly memories "come back." I can walk along a street and know, without searching my memory, the name of the next street; I can pick up a phone and dial a number I did not "know" for years. Lost memories need not reflect repression, nor does their recovery necessarily indicate a breaking down of repressive, defensive barriers; it may as well indicate the reinstatement of an earlier context.

In the concept being developed here, early emotional experiences are seen as important but by no means exclusive determinants of adult functioning, nor does therapeutic change depend on discovering their original nature. Even if a particular facet of personality is clearly rooted in traumatic or conflict-laden early experiences, subsequent change can occur without necessarily bringing those experiences to light. Neurotic patterns are rooted in the past, but they are sustained through present forces.

Historical events, therefore, are to be studied from the vantage point of the contemporary personality. What matters most is how such events are remembered and how the patient now understands them; what actually occurred in the past and what meaning it had then we may be able to infer but that is of lesser importance. Thus, the patient who felt rejected on his first day on the new job, may report that his parents "always" favored his older brother, and treated him as an unworthy and unlovable appendage to the family. He recalls incidents showing how he was neglected and he feels again the resulting hurt. Today, he still resents his brother and his parents and he cannot relate to them without angry feelings, not however unmixed with envy and a plaintive hope that they will come to appreciate and love him. His readiness to expect social rebuff may be a generalized expectation derived from his sense of unworthiness in the earlier family constellation. In further exploration of early memories, the patient may recall incidents in which he was treated with loving consideration. The patient may dismiss such incidents as atypical, but the therapist can use them to challenge his "always" concept. However, what is ultimately needed is a break in the belief system- "I am an unworthy little boy and people have always and will always treat me as insignificant and unlovable." In therapy, this may occur as a consequence of one or more of the following conditions: (I) The patient recovers hitherto repressed feelings and memories which can be relived in the present therapeutic relationship; (2) He can reconceptualize earlier experiences, whether repressed, distorted, or accurately remembered. ("Yes, I guess there were other times when I was treated fairly," or more radically, "Whatever happened in the past, I can now lead a new life."); or (3) He can be encouraged to discover new, relevant sources of competence and worth in his present life, including importantly the therapeutic relation itself which gives immediate and living evidence of his worth. While all of these processes may occur, the third is ultimately the most important for producing the corrective emotional experiences of therapy.

Exploring the Therapist-patient Relationship

The relation between the therapist and the patient sets the basic emotional climate within which the patient is willing to undertake self-exploration. In the on-going process of psychotherapy, the relation serves three further functions, as it provides (I) a microcosm of social behavior generally; (2) an opportunity for examining transference feelings; and (3) an opportunity for learning through identification and modeling.

Microcosm of other social relations However special the transactions between patient and therapist, in some respects it is like other social relations in the patient's life. Behavior varies in different social roles, hence the patient-therapist interplay is predictably different from, for example, the patient-spouse or patient (as student)-teacher interactions. Still, there are consistencies across roles which reflect personality traits. Thus, the submissive person hesitates to express opinions to his spouse, to his teacher and to his therapist, while the assertive person is more ready to speak his mind to all three. Hence, while a considerable part of therapy focuses on events occurring outside of the session, there is in the session itself a constant, on-going flow between the two participants within which the patient, and so too the therapist, reveal characteristic interpersonal attitudes. The immediate information contained in the here-and-now situations of therapy therefore provides a framework for understanding the patient's problems and personality. They provide illustrations of more or less typical behaviors, against which the patient's descriptions of "life" behaviors can be viewed. Thus, the patient who says "I always stutter when I talk about myself," yet at the moment is speaking with perfect clarity. This contradiction can be called to his attention. Either he exaggerates the extent of his distress or it occurs only when speaking with certain kinds of people in some kinds of situations; whatever the case, the present behavior gives context for understanding outside behavior. In addition, of considerable importance are those feelings directed toward the therapist himself as the relation develops. The patient can feel resentment, affection, dependence, respect, or any of numerous other feelings which are more or less appropriate and predictable in such an intimate situation.

The role of transference feelings. Among the reactions to the therapist are those which Freud described as "transference." These are attitudes carried over from early experiences which are now projected onto the therapist, who has not, so to speak, earned them himself. While one might readily feel warmly respectful toward a kind and wise therapist, and even wish to have further contact with him as a friend, it is inappropriate to feel intense love and to yearn for a sexual relationship. Such feelings, psychoanalysts propose, are carry-overs from blocked needs in early life, particularly in relation to one's own parents. The analysis of transference feelings is of central importance to the psychoanalytic process for they bring into present consciousness critical, usually repressed, conflicts of the past. It should be noted that the conditions of psychoanalytic therapy, such as frequent sessions over a long period, encouragement of unconscious fantasy, and the impersonality of the therapist, particularly encourage the development of transference. However, the phenomenon of transferred or projected feelings occurs in any form of therapy and the therapist should be prepared for the onslaught of feelings which are disproportionate to present realities. So too, the good therapist has to be able to distinguish "earned" from "transferred" feelings and know his own contribution to the patient's state. If I yawn repeatedly as the patient talks about matters of great importance to him and he then tells me that I must think him unworthy of my concern, it is at least insensitive to suggest that he is recalling his sense of inferiority in the presence of his father. The fact is that I yawned, which correctly enough he can interpret as boredom, and that fact has to be faced first. The line between realistic, appropriate feelings anchored in the present encounter and unrealistic, exaggerated feelings rooted in historically determined neurotic needs of the patient is surely a difficult one to draw. Both types of feelings are important in therapy; transference reactions, however, have the special quality of revealing what may be critically important and deeply rooted attitudes toward major figures in the patient's earlier life.

Learning through identification and modeling. The relation between therapist and patient figures in still another way in psychotherapy. It provides opportunity for the patient to observe and take on the behaviors of the therapist through an identification and/or modeling process. Bandura has called particular attention to the importance of modeling, particularly when working with children. However, in all forms of therapeutic intervention, patients tend to adopt the therapist's ways of thinking, feeling, and acting, sometimes by intent but as often unwittingly through a process of identification and internalization. This may be seen in trivial and not particularly desirable ways, as for example by the patient taking on the therapist's mannerisms or taste in clothing. Some finish therapy not much changed except for a Van Dyke beard, tweedy sport coat, and saying "So?" with a slightly Viennese accent. The gain is more substantial, however, if the patient has learned to plan actions instead of acting impulsively, to remain calm under stress, and to face his own inadequacies rather than denying them, in part at least inspired by observing these qualities in his therapist.

Recognizing, Clarifying and Interpreting Patient's Feelings and Meanings

The therapist listens intently and at various times offers interpretive comments on what the patient says. Through these interjections, the therapist calls attention to the patient's feelings and beliefs, identifies and clarifies them, puts them into the context of other aspects of his personality, fosters awareness of their possible antecedents, and ultimately, one hopes, provides opportunity for the patient to alter his behavior in terms of the increased self-awareness. Interpretation focuses both on the what and the why of behavior, in order to increase awareness of what the patient is presently feeling and what impact it may have on others and as well as to discover why, in terms of the patient's needs, character structure, and determining experiences, he has come to feel, believe, or act in this particular way. In general, in the earlier stages of the therapy process emphasis is on what and only later on why. Whatever their focus, and however simple or complex, the intended effect of interpretation is to alter the patient's cognitions of himself and his world.

At the simplest level, interpretations may involve repeating or restating something the patient has said, perhaps altering the emphasis, to make him more aware of its import. Thus, in reply to the patient's "Nothing went right today," the therapist might reply

"Nothing?" Even the simple "Tell me more," carries the meaning that the issue is important and more information desirable. More complex interpretations, involving increasing degrees of inference, include those which attempt to identify and name the feeling state behind the patient's comments, those which summarize a number of parallel productions in order to draw attention to common themes, and those which call to the patient's awareness attitudes of which he seems unaware or may actively be denying. Illustrative interpretive comments in these modes might include: "You seem to be very angry when you talk about him." "It seems that when you get into a frustrating situation, you feel like quitting and giving up." "You say you respect him, but I keep hearing you make disparaging remarks about him." Still more complex and inferential are those interpretations which attempt to show linkages between the patient's feelings toward important figures of the past and those in his current life, including the therapist himself (transference reactions). Finally, there are those interpretations directed toward possible symbolic meanings or theoretical constructs.

The concept of interpretation originates in psychoanalysis, where it usually refers to the more complex forms of inferences, particularly those which seek to explain current personality characteristics in terms of repressed and unconscious conflicts and needs. Classically the effort was directed at divining ultimate causes of the patient's symptoms in terms of their originating experiences. Interpretation is now made of defensive strategies, resistance, and transference reactions in therapy, and of current fantasies, impulses, and behavior, not only to discover their origins but to understand their dynamics in contemporary functioning. Thus, Fromm-Reichmann states:

> *The purpose of interpretation and of interpretive questions is to bring dissociated and repressed experiences and motivations to awareness and to show patients how, unknown to themselves, repressed and dissociated material finds its expression in and colors verbalized communications and behavior patterns such as their actions, attitudes, and gestures.*

The concept of interpretation as used here is intended in a broader meaning, not limited to discovering and revealing "dissociated and repressed experiences and motivations," whether in a historic or contemporary framework. Rather the term, it seems to me, can properly be used to describe any intentional act by the therapist which attempts to foster understanding by calling attention to unknown or ignored factors, by bringing together hitherto unrelated materials and by proposing explanations for feelings and actions, whether or not in terms of unconscious determinants. Thus, included would be "recognizing and clarifying feelings" in the sense used by Carl Rogers, who properly describes his psychotherapy as "noninterpretive" when the term is limited to the psychoanalytic usage. While it might be well to use several terms to describe different levels, complexity, and targets of interpretive acts, they all have in common the effort to reconceptualize the meanings of the patient's communications.

In this conception, therapeutic interpretation can be visualized as ranging from lower-order judgments of a simple, more descriptive type to higher-order inferences of a more conceptual or abstract nature, along much the same type of continuum previously used to describe the interpretive acts of clinical assessment. Viewed in terms of the clinician's thought processes, interpreting the "data" of therapeutic encounters and those of assessment interviews and tests are quite analogous enterprises. Both require careful observation and disciplined clinical judgment, anchored in extensive knowledge of personality mechanisms and theory. In both cases, there must be a blending of inferential and intuitive processes; on the one hand, the painstaking gathering, processing and generalization of relevant information and on the other, the use of creative imagination and divergent thinking required to create as well as to test hypotheses. In both cases, judgment can be flawed by the operation of many factors, such as schematization, lack of individualization, over interpretation, and the like considered earlier.

There are, of course, critical differences between interpretation in assessment and in therapy. In assessment, standardized procedures can be used for which there are norms and hence opportunity for statistical inference. Moreover, the clinician has all his material before him, which he can study and restudy and as necessary gather further information before reaching conclusions. In therapy, by contrast, he is in the midst of a flowing stream and interpretive comments have to be made with minimum forethought.

But, by the same token, the clinician is dealing with decidedly smaller units at each moment. Moreover, should he miss one opportunity, there are repeated occasions to call attention to the same theme. Most important is the fact that in therapy the clinician has immediate feedback and, by virtue of the therapeutic alliance, collaboration in judging the patient's productions. The patient's immediate reaction advises the therapist as to the credibility of the interpretation and guides his further comments. The patient not only responds to the therapist's interpretations, but he himself actively generates hypotheses about his behavior.

Much has been written about the correctness of interpretation, but the issue is more the plausibility and working value of the interpretation, rather than its literal truth. They are hypotheses as to what is going on; the best guess under the circumstances and they are meant to be tentatively held and considered. They are valuable to the extent that they define issues and move the therapeutic dialogue forward. A gratifying response is "you know, I never thought of it that way, maybe that's why ..." or "I've been thinking about what you said last week and I decided to try it out by acting differently with my wife." Rarely if ever does a single interpretation, or even a series over time, lead to a radical reconceptualization of the patient's problem in a blinding flash of insight.

Interpretations achieve a number of effects in addition to facilitating the recognition, clarification, and understanding of the patient's feelings. They imply acceptance or rejection of the patient's concerns. Labeling a feeling state, for example, reveals to the patient that the feeling is acceptable to the therapist, though the patient may have felt that he would be repelled by it. On the other hand, interpretations suggesting the inappropriateness or maladaptive nature of some act imply criticism and suggest directions for change. Correspondingly, interpretations can alter the patient's emotional state as wall as rousing specific affects. Some interpretations increase the patient's sense of mastery or his faith in the therapist and lead to a reduction of tension; others reveal his inadequacies or bring into view hitherto unknown fantasies or feelings and heighten distress.

Thus, a patient can feel more guilty at the realization that he holds feelings more vicious than he had imagined, but again a patient's guilt might be alleviated by the discovery that others share such feelings. Finally, it should be noted that interpretations convey a conceptual scheme for understanding one's own and the behavior of others. At the very least, the patient comes to understand that behavior is explicable and hence meaningful, even when seemingly determined by powerful forces beyond his understanding and control.

Early in therapy, the therapist focuses mainly on clarifying present feelings and attitudes as they are immediately revealed in the sessions. Much of the emphasis is on his current concerns including his motivation for therapy. Only later are more far-reaching interpretations possible. This is partly because more information is needed of the sort which emerges only with time and growing confidence in the therapist. Moreover, a firm relation is needed to absorb the potentially damaging effects of an inept or inopportune interpretation. The higher the level of inference involved, the greater is the risk that the interpretation will be erroneous and be more painful than helpful to the patient. Too often, interpretations offered seem more intended to show off the therapist's intellectual agility at contriving an all-inclusive view of the patient in favored theoretical terms, than to organize the experiences of the patient in ways meaningful to him. Harry Stack Sullivan, the eminently sensitive and sensible interpersonal psychiatrist, cautioned his students that "The supply of interpretations, like that of advice, greatly exceeds the need for them." .In his own work, he tried to understand the patient as if from inside and generally limited his comments to those most likely to make the patient more fully aware of what he was actually experiencing.

In general, interpretative comments should be close to where the patient is at in his evolving self-awareness. Though few general rules can be made, it seems true that an interpretation is most effective when it anticipates, but not by much, an emerging consciousness of an issue; when a notion is, as it were, on the tip of the patient's mental tongue but not yet consciously available. It is all too easy to know after the fact when an interpretive comment misfires or is premature, or even when it has been delayed too long, but to know the opportune moment as it arises is one of the most difficult tasks of the psychotherapist. One thing is certain, however, just because a hypothesis occurs to the therapist is no reason for him to immediately verbalize it to the patient. Most often such interpretations are simply to be held in mind, developed in the therapist's thinking as more evidence cumulates, and offered to the patient only when the time seems right for him to absorb and use it. In the ensuing dialogue, the ramifications and value of the hypothesis are tested conjointly with the patient, toward the end of extending, altering, or rejecting it as necessary. Although there are dramatic accounts of important symptoms of psychological changes following interpretive acts even in a single interview, much more usually, the linked processes of examining experience, seeking relations, and offering and testing clarificatory concepts require numerous therapeutic transactions in which many of the same issues are discussed repeatedly, if from differing points of view.

From Understanding to Action

In general terms, psychotherapy can be viewed as consisting of three major phases: (1) Establishing the therapeutic relationship, with the necessary motivation and trust, fundamental commitment and therapeutic alliance, and a workable contract from which therapy can proceed; (2) Seeking understanding of the nature and sources of personality characteristics and defects. This is the major task of therapy and typically involves relentless examination and interpretation of current feelings, attitudes, and behaviors and their historical antecedents and of the patient's relation with relevant others, including the therapist; and (3)Translating insights into actions and new life patterns. Failure can occur at any level, but if successful, the patient passes through all three. Thus far, we have considered the first two stages; at this point let us look at the third.

The self-knowledge of the second phase is painfully and arduously, if at all, won. Nor can progress be plotted on a smooth, ascending curve. There are setbacks as new problems arise, life conditions change, or the patient meets defeats in halting efforts at more positive behaviors. Neurotic patterns are not easily shed and patients move back to safer ground after seeming advances. Hence, there is constant need to reexamine, reinterpret, and reanalyze emotional patterns, time and again, in order to consolidate the gains of earlier therapeutic dialogues. This process has been called "working through" and it merges with the more positive activities of the third phase. However, to the extent that the patient has discovered underlying patterns in his behavior, has greater understanding of what he does and to an extent why, and has become aware of the functional roles played by out-moded and self-defeating defenses and character traits, dissatisfaction with them grows apace and with it resolve to change and willingness to try new behaviors. With self-awareness, there is an increased sense of emotional security, self-esteem, and mastery. The patient is more ready to discard old habits and values and to experiment with new actions; he has been liberated to seek more autonomous and constructive behaviors. Throughout, but particularly in this phase, as the patient has been able to master emotional conflicts in the therapeutic relation, he can venture out to try his new skills in "real life." As Alexander put it:

> *Like the adage "Nothing succeeds like success," there is no more powerful therapeutic factor than the performance of activities which were formerly neurotically impaired or inhibited. No insight, no emotional discharge, no recollection can be as reassuring as accomplishment in the actual life situation in which the individual failed. Thus the ego regains that confidence which is the fundamental condition, the prerequisite, of mental health. Every success encourages new trials and decreases inferiority feelings, resentments, and their sequelae-fear, guilt, and resulting inhibitions. Successful attempts at productive work, love, self-assertion, or competition will change the vicious circle to a benign one; as they are repeated, they become habitual and thus eventually bring about a complete change in the personality.*

In the third and last phase, therapeutic conversations generally turn from (1) consideration of neurotic patterns to discussion of adaptive potentials; (2) inner feelings, fantasies, and memories to outside social realities; and (3) from past history and present problems to future prospects. In fair measure, the basic activity of therapy continues, that is, the patient talks about his concerns and the therapist attempts to clarify and advance understanding. However, there are important changes in the therapy process. The relation between therapist and patient becomes more that of equals. The patient has learned a therapeutic mode of thinking and he is more likely to volunteer interpretations, introduce topics, pose questions and seek advice. As emotional tensions are reduced, he is able to reason more logically. Freer of neurotic resistances and defenses, he can more readily formulate, and is more open to accept, alternate interpretations of his behavior. Increasingly, therefore, the therapist and patient are partners in a joint problem solving task.

On his part, the therapist paradoxically is freer to act in more directive ways. He can encourage specific actions, offer direct advice, suggest one rather than another alternative. Earlier in therapy such interventions are avoided lest the patient passively obey out of excessive fear, dependence, or awe. But once the patient is better able to make up his own mind, and defend his own positions, the therapist is able to state his own more positively. Where earlier persuasive efforts might seem manipulations of the patient's weakness, they are now more tributes to his strength. Consequently, the therapist can urge particular actions and openly compliment or criticize his efforts. This is not at all to suggest that the therapist has given up the investigatory role in favor of a directive one; major effort still goes into trying to discover the meanings of the patient's wishes and actions. But now, meanings can be tested against direct as well as more indirect reactions. The apparently simple statement "Why do you think that will work?" should now draw from the patient "for the following reasons, a...b...c...," whereas it might have evoked "maybe I better not try ..." earlier. In this phase, too, there is need to encourage exploratory activities in previously avoided realms. To this end, supportive encouragement can be valuable without being coercive.

With the patient directing more attention to future activities in the outside world, the therapist can facilitate decision making by vicariously testing alternative possibilities with him. "Well, suppose you went back to school ... how would that affect your way of life ... relations with friends ... your wife ... etc. ?" "If you go into business for yourself, you would have more independence to run things your way, but you'd have less free time ... more responsibility ... maybe less income, at first at least? Are you willing to make the trade off?" In some ways, the task is more like that of a psychological consultant facilitating the rational decision-making of an executive than that of a therapist disentangling the confused emotions of a distressed person. Role playing may be a valuable technique for discovering what may be involved in a hitherto untried social situation. Thus, if the patient is fearful at the prospect of a job interview, he and the therapist can enact the roles of applicant and personnel man. In the course of the pretended job interview, the patient reveals his expectations, how he would present himself, his ways of acting, reacting to challenges, and the like. The therapist meanwhile can by playing his role in different ways more or less vigorously test the patient. At the end, they can examine the episode together toward discovering ways in which the patient might improve his chances in a future real-life job interview. Similarly, the therapist might assist the patient frame a letter of application, review with him information on the job market, help him focus vocational or educational goals, or otherwise help him find a more satisfying place for increased talents and personality resources.

Terminating Psychotherapy

A cynic has said that psychotherapy ends when the patient becomes as bored listening to himself as the therapist has been all along. Actually, there is a partial truth here. It is a sign of health for a patient to become less consumed with his problems, to see them as more manageable and less important, and hence to prefer putting his energies into seeking new experiences rather than in licking old wounds. The error lies in the implication that the patient was all along self-indulgently dwelling on trivial matters, which depreciates both his pain and the therapist's potential contribution to its relief.

When should psychotherapy end? In one sense, never. There is no limit to personal development and hence therapy, in the essential meaning of the conscious examination, understanding, and perfecting of behavior, is similarly a life long process. Psychotherapy is a desirable way of life, which may but does not necessarily involve more than one's own efforts within a therapeutic way of thinking. Such a therapeutic attitude, though a natural part of mature behavior, can be learned in sessions with a professional, and then hopefully carried over to guide future life.

In the more usual and limited sense, psychotherapy should be terminated when the stated goals are reached. The more precisely these were originally phrased, the more certain therapist and patient can be that they have been attained. Thus, we can know with some certainty that presenting symptoms have disappeared or that work can be resumed, but with decidedly less confidence that the patient has developed "emotional maturity" or "resources for creative living." Moreover, new vistas open and goals change as therapy progresses; also, therapist and patient may all along have had different notions of what was expected at the end. Whatever the case, however, the terminal phase necessarily begins with therapist and patient taking stock of the patient's current status and future prospects and deciding whether goals are closely enough approached.

With this decision it is well to set a particular final date, approximately six weeks later, and even to taper off in the final weeks by reducing the frequency or length of sessions. Emphasis in this phase is on the meaning of discontinuing therapy as well as on the patient's plans for the future. There are predictable emotional problems which may have to be dealt with. Just as there are resistances to making commitments to the therapy in the first place, there can be resistances to leaving it at the end. For some patients, being in therapy becomes a way of life, rather than a proper means to an end. Though completing therapy is an achievement, and betokens movement to a more mature level of self-management, it may still be experienced as rejection. There is often a surge of dependent feelings. The patient is suddenly afraid to venture out on his own, and "Wouldn't a few more sessions help ... ?" There may be a resurgence of earlier symptoms, as if to prove the point, or just generalized distress and anxiety. In some ways, the situation is not unlike the adolescent who may have been rebelliously proclaiming his right to autonomy and yet feels strangely fearful as he leaves the family for college. Uncertainty is an understandable enough feeling when one moves from one life phase to another, but so too is excitement and hope. The effort in the last phase is to accentuate the latter and minimize the former feelings. It is important to assure the patient that, if there are setbacks in the future, additional sessions can be scheduled, even if expressing the hope that they will not be needed.

It is a paradox of psychotherapy that it is a dependent relation-the patient seeks and obtains "help"-the goal of which is independent functioning. In the nondirective mode described in this chapter, the patient is given maximal respect and autonomy throughout and he collaborates with increasing responsibility in the process. Hence, the transition to still greater freedom after therapy should be, and usually is, an occasion for joy. In more directive modes, which build on the patient's dependency, termination can be a harsher experience. However, in this or any form of psychotherapy, problems of the type discussed can arise in the final weeks. Indeed, it is a measure of the success of psychotherapy that the patient can move smoothly into an autonomous life in which he is, so to speak, his own therapist. Termination is, as graduation speakers remind us, a "commencement," the beginning of a new and better era.

Termination of course can, and often does, occur before goals are reached and with little or no sense of accomplishment. Therapy may have come to an impasse and with the best efforts of patient and therapist, all that can be visualized is a long and futile plateau. Despite earlier resolve, the patient may now be confronting neurotic mechanisms which he cannot or will not change. On the other hand, the patient may terminate therapy "prematurely" because he feels his goals have been reached, even though it may seem obvious to the therapist or onlooker that there are still many outstanding problems. Earlier, note was taken of the fact that therapists not infrequently expect more for their patients than do the patients themselves. From the patient's view, therefore, termination in such cases may not be at all premature. In research on the outcome of therapy the patient's unilateral decision to discontinue is often taken as a sign of failure, when actually it may be success from the patient's point of view. However, walking out in anger or disgust, with a sense of futility and that time and effort were wasted, is another matter. Still, even under these circumstances, the decision to quit sometimes leads to reconsideration and recommitment to therapy.

A funny-sad illustration concerns an old friend who, though a competent professional, was an impulsive, readily arousable person with little tolerance of disappointment or delay. Impatient with the plodding pace of therapy, he simply announced one day that he'd had enough, without failing, however, to accuse his therapist of incompetence. The therapist's last words, as my friend left, were "Please be careful going home." To celebrate his new-found freedom and wealth, now that he would no longer be paying for therapy, he decided to stop and buy glasses and dishes to replace his old mismatched and chipped ones. Loosely wrapped bags were put on the back seat and he took off for home. Only a few blocks later, he carelessly ran into the rear of a car at a stoplight, dumping his glasses and dishes all over himself and the floor of the car. He showed up at the time of the next scheduled therapy session contrite and now ready to get down to work.

Therapy may also be discontinued because the therapist feels that he is no longer capable of working with the patient. Either he recognizes that he lacks sufficient knowledge, experience, or skill to treat this particular kind of patient or problem or he discovers that he has lost the necessary therapeutic detachment by developing overly strong personal feelings, some of which reflect counter transference in the psychoanalytic sense. Just as the patient can project onto the therapist out-moded and inappropriate attitudes, the therapist can do the same to the patient. Such feelings may also be stimulated by salient qualities of the patient, who may, in fact, hold despicable social attitudes or be extraordinarily attractive.

In principle, the well-disciplined therapist should have sufficient self-knowledge, control, and tolerance to continue with this patient despite the arousal of hate or lust. Such feelings can be honestly discussed with the patient, or to advantage reviewed with a colleague or supervisor, but if they become sufficiently demanding, termination may be the only responsible solution. If therapy is discontinued because of the therapist's inadequacies, he has a special obligation to make this clear to the patient, lest the patient be left with a sense of guilt and the feeling that he is a hopeless case. Wherever appropriate, effort should be made to help him find another therapist.

Finally, therapy can be brought to an end for adventitious reasons. The patient or therapist may have to move from the area or one or the other may become too ill to continue. Jobs can change, and the patient may not be able to schedule the therapy hours; perhaps his new position requires him to travel continuously. In training clinics, psychotherapy is usually limited to the academic year, at the end of which student clinicians move on to new assignments. Under all such circumstances, therapy should be brought to as useful a close as possible. Even if not a natural ending point, the last weeks can be used profitably in reviewing the progress and status of the patient, considering the import of termination, and planning for the future.

Bibliography

Anderson N. *The hobo; the sociology of the homeless man*. Chicago: Univ. of Chicago Press, 1923.

Andrew, Gwen, Walton, R. E., Hartwell, S. W., and Hutt M. The Michigan picture test: The stimulus values of the cards. *J. consult. Psychol.*, 1951, 15, 51-54.

Androp S. Electric shock therapy in psychoses; convulsive and subconvulsive methods. *Psychiat. Quart.*, 1941, 15, 730-749.

Baker, H. J., and Traphagen V. *The Detroit scale for the diagnosis of behavior problems*. New York: Macmillan, 1935.

Balken, E. R., and Masserman, J. H. "The language of phantasy: III. The language of the phantasies of patients with conversion hysteria, anxiety state, and obsessive-compulsive neuroses." *J. Psychol.*, 1940, 10, 75-86.

Balken, E. R., and Vander Veer, A. H. "The clinical application of a test of imagination to neurotic children." *Amer. J. Orthopsychiat.*, 1942, 12, 68-80.

Champney H. "The measurement of parent behavior." *Child. Develpm.*, 1941, 12, 131-166.

Cheney C. O. (Ed.). *Outlines of psychiatric examinations*. Utica, N.Y.: State Hospitals Press, 1934.

Clark M. A. "Directory of psychiatric clinics in the United States, 1936". *Ment. Hyg.*, 1936, 20, 66-129.

Dennis W. "The effect of cradling practices upon the onset of walking in Hopi children". *J. genet. Psychol.*, 1940, 56, 77-86.

Deri Susan K. "Description of the Szondi test: a projective technique for psychological diagnosis". *Amer. Psychologist,* 1946, 1, 239. (Abstract.)

Deri Susan K. *Introduction to the Szondi test.* New York: Grune & Stratton, 1949.

Dunlap K. *Habits: their making and unmaking.* New York: Liveright, 1933.

Dussik K. T., and Sakel M. "*Ergebnisse der Hypoglykamie-schockbehandlung der Schizophrenia*". *Z. ges. Neurol. Psychiat.,* 1936, 155, 351-415.

Ebaugh F. G. "Association-motor investigation in clinical psychiatry". *J. ment. Sci.,* 1936, 82, 731-743.

Edwards A. L., and Kenney Kathryn C. "A comparison of the Thurstone and Likert techniques of attitude scale construction". *2J. appl. Psychol.,* 1946, 30, 72-83.

Esquirol J.-E. D. *Des maladies mentales considérées sous les rapports médical, hygiénique, et médico-légal. Paris: J. C. Baillière, 1838. Vols. I, II, and Atlas. (Not seen.)*

Eysenck H. J. "Training in clinical psychology: An English point of view". *Amer. Psychologist,* 1949, 4, 173-176.

Farrell M. J., and Vassaf E. "Effect of insulin shock on heart and blood pressure in treatment of schizophrenia". *Arch. Neurol. Psychiat.,* 1940, 43, 784-791.

Flanagan J. C. *Factor analysis in the study of personality.* Stanford Univ., Calif.: Stanford Univ. Press, 1935.

Flescher J. Sulla "funzione di discorcia" dell elettroshock ed il problema dell "ansia." *Psychoanalisi,* 1946, 2, 85-89.

Fonda C. P. "The nature and meaning of the Rorschach white space response". *J. abnorm. soc. Psychol.,* 1951, 46, 367-377.

Gellhorn E., Kessler M., and Minatoya H. "Influence of metrazol, insulin hypoglycemia and electrically induced convulsions on reestablishment of inhibited conditioned reflexes". *Proc. Soc. exp. Biol. Med.,* 1942, 50, 260262.

Gesell A. *Infancy and human growth.* New York: Macmillan, 1928.

Gibbs F. A., Davis H., and Lennox W. G. The electroencephalogram in epilepsy and in conditions of impaired consciousness . *Arch. Neurol. Psychiat.,* Chicago, 1935, 34, 1133-1148.

Harris A. J., and Shakow D. "Scatter on the Stanford-Binet in schizophrenic, normal, and delinquent adults". *J. abnorm. soc. Psychol.*, 1938, 33, 100-111.

Harris R. E., Bowman K. M., and Simon A. "Studies in electronarcoses therapy. III. Psychological test findings". *J. nerv. ment. Dis.*, 1948, 107, 371-376.

Harris W. W. "A bas-relief projective technique". *J. Psychol.*, 1948, 26, 3-17.

Jennings Helen H. Structure of leadership-development and sphere of influence. *Sociometry*, 1937, 1, 99-143.

Jervis G. A. The genetics of phenylpyruvic oligophrenia. *Proc. Amer. Ass. ment. Def.*, 1938- 1939, 44, 13-24.

Jessner Lucie and Ryan V. G. *Shock treatment in psychiatry*. New York: Grune & Stratton, 1941.

Jolliffe N. Treatment of neuro-psychiatric disorders with vitamins. *S. Amer. med. Ass.*, 1941, 117, 1496- 1502.

Kanner L. *Child psychiatry*. Springfield, Ill.: Charles C Thomas, 1935.

Larrabee H. A. *Reliable knowledge*. Boston: Houghton Mifflin, 1945.

Lashley K. S. *Brain mechanisms and intelligence, a quantitative study of injuries to the brain*. Chicago: Univ. of Chicago Press, 1929.

Lazarsfeld P. F., and ROBINSON W. S. The quantification of case studies. *J. appl. Psychol.*, 1940, 24, 817-825.

Lazarus R. S. The influence of color on the protocol of the Rorschach test. *J. abnorm. soc. Psychol.*, 1949, 44, 506-516.

Lazarus R. S., Deese J. E., and Osler Sonia F. The effects of psychological stress upon performance. *Psychol. Bull.*, 1952. (In press.)

Machover Karen. *Personality projection in the drawing of the human figure*. Springfield, Ill.: Charles C Thomas, 1948.

Mackinnon D. W. The structure of personality. In J. McV. HUNT (Ed.), *Personality and the behavior disorders*. New York: Ronald, 1944.

Malinowski B. *Crime and custom in savage society*. New York: Harcourt, Brace, 1926.

Mckinney F. Directive techniques. In L. A. and I. A. Berg Pennington (Eds.), *An introduction to clinical psychology*. New York: Ronald, 1948.

McNemar Q. *The revision of the Stanford-Binet scale.* Boston: Houghton Mifflin, 1942.

Norbury F. G. " Applications of Vitamin B to neuropsychiatry". *Ill. med. Soc.,* 1940, 78, 228-232.

Peterson J. *Early conceptions and tests of intelligence.* Yonkers, N.Y.: World, 1925.

Rabin A. I. "Differentiating psychometric patterns in schizophrenia and manicdepressive psychosis". *J. abnorm. soc. Psychol.,* 1942, 37, 270-272.

Rabin A. I. "Test score patterns in schizophrenia and non-psychotic states". *Psychol.,* 1941, 12, 91-100.

Sarason S. B., and Rosenzweig S. "An experimental study of the triadic hypothesis: reaction to frustration, ego-defense, and hypnotizability. II. Thematic apperception approach". *Character & Pers.,* 1942, 11, 150-165.

Sargent H. "Projective methods: their origins, theory and application in personality research". *Psychol. Bull.,* 1945, 42, 257-293.

Thorndike E. L. *The Institute of Educational Research intelligence scale CAVD.* New York: Bureau of Publications, Teachers College, Columbia Univ., 1925.

Wertheimer M. "Studies in the theory of Gestalt psychology." *Psychol. Forsch.,* 1923, 4, 300-350.

Whipple G. M. "Tests of imagination and invention, Test 45, ink-blots." In G. M. WHIPPLE, *Manual of mental and physical tests.* Baltimore: Warwick and York, 1910.

White R. R. "Influence of suggestibility on responses in ink spot tests." *Child Develpm.,* 1931, 2, 76-79.

INDEX

V

W